HOME LEG WORKOUTS FOR WOMEN

One-Minute Moves To Help You Get Leaner, Stronger, Faster

by Amber O'Connor

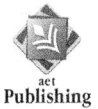

aet
Publishing

All Rights Reserved. No part of this publication may be reproduced in any form or by any means, including scanning, photocopying, or otherwise without prior written permission of the copyright holder.

Copyright © 2014 AET Publishing
Cover Art and Interior Artwork by Gracie .K. Jones

ISBN-10: 1502526484

Website:
www.oneminutemovesbooks.com

Mobile site:
m.oneminutemovesbooks.com

Pinterest:
pinterest.com/ommbooks

Are You Getting The Right Balance?

Want to feel more upbeat, have more energy and better concentration? Maybe you also want to lose a few pounds? Then it's time you took a realistic look at your diet and lifestyle.

To see if your lifestyle could be affecting your health, take this quick quiz at http://www.oneminutemovesbooks.com/quiz

Section One: Introduction 10

Why Lower Body Strength Training is Important 10
    The Benefits You Gain From Strength Training 11
    The EPOC Boost: The Post Exercise Fat Sizzler for Added Weight Loss 11
    What's in This Book? 11

Section Two: Basic Stretching 13

Creating Your Own Basic Stretching Routine 13

Ankle Flex 14

Toe Balances 15

Standing Calf Stretches 16

Quad Stretch 17

Inner Thigh Stretch 18

Lying Piriformis Stretch (for Rotator Muscles) 19

Standing Hamstring Stretch 20

Shin and Ankle Stretches 21

Standing Full Body Stretch 22
    Learn How to Stretch in 3 Moves 23

Back Stretch on Fitness Ball 24

Lying Leg Extensions 25

Power Skips 26

Hip Swings 27

Straight Leg Kicks 28

High Knees 29

Marching on the Spot 30

Section Three: Beginners Workouts 31

Basic Lower Body Exercise Guidelines for Beginners 32
    Some General Workout Tips 32

1. One Leg Balance 34

2. Table Top Balance on Fitness Ball 35

3. Side Step-outs with Knee Raise 36

4. Step-ups with Arm Raises 37

5. Inner Thigh Lifts 38

6. Outer Thigh Lifts 39
   Is Spot Reduction Fact or Fiction? 40

7. Hip Lifts 41

8. Frog Hops 42

9. Plies 44

10. Calf Raises 45

Section Four: Glutes, Hips and Thighs Workouts 46

The Slow Burn: Why Lower Body Fat is Hard to Shift for Women 46
   3 Tips to Help Your Hips, Glutes and Thighs Win the War Against Biology (and Gravity) 47

11. Forward Lunges 49
    Why Forward Lunges Are Great For Glutes and Thighs 49

12. Side Kick Squats 51

13. Knee thrust to Front Kick 53

14. Side Kicks 55

15. Kickbacks 56

16. Kickbacks with Resistance Band 57

17. One Legged Squats 58

18. Shoulder Width Squats 59

19. Dead Lifts 60

Section Five: Fitness Ball Workouts 61

More Toning Power in Less Time: Why You Get Faster Results Using a Fitness Ball 61
   How to Pick the Best Fitness Ball for Your Home Workouts 62

20. Lying Hamstring Curl 63

21. *Sitting Knee Lifts 64*

22. *Standing Knee Lifts 65*
    Why Exercise Balls are a Winner for Functional Fitness 67

23. *Bridge 68*

24. *Standing Leg Swings/Kicks 69*

25. *Sitting Walks 70*

26. *Spilt Squats 71*

27. *Wall Squats 72*

28. *Single Leg Wall Squats 73*

29. *Leg Presses 74*

30. *Supported Lean Back 75*

Section Six: Body-weight Workouts 76

Benefits of Body-weight Exercises 76
Train on One, Rule on Two: Building Stronger Limbs with Single Leg Exercises 76

31. *Jump Squats 78*
    Getting the Most Out of Your Body-Weight Exercises 79

32. *Standing Knee Hug 80*

33. *Side Knee Hug 81*

34. *Front and Side Swings 82*
    How to Accelerate Fat Loss with Body-Weight Moves 83
    5 MRT Tricks to Help You Boost Post Workout Fat Burn 83

35. *Prisoner Cycle Lunge 84*

36. *Ski Moguls 86*

37. *Single Leg Heel Raises 87*

Section Seven: Floor Workouts 88

Pilates: The Ultimate 'Squat Free' Floor Workout for Sculpting Legs 88
The Core Connection: How Using Your Abs Benefits Your Lower Body 88

38. *Adductor Squeeze 90*

39. *Crossed Legged Bridge 91*

40. Single Leg Circles 92

41. Single Leg Kick 93

42. Swimming 94

43. Bird-Dog 95

44. Single Leg Stretch 96

45. Hip Raise/Glute Bridge 97

Section Eight: Knee Strengthening Workouts 98

Knee Anatomy 101 98
    Why Stronger Thighs Equals Stronger Knees 98
    Why Better Flexibility Also Means Stronger Knees 99

46. Tree Pose 101

47. Bridge with Straight Leg Raise 102

48. Warrior II 103

49. Modified Side Angle Pose 104

50. Standing Knee Bends (Shallow Squats) 105

51. The Plank 107
    6 Ways to Keep Your Knees Healthy 108

52. Prone Plank 110

53. Standing Cradle Leg Stretch 111

Section Nine: Pregnancy Leg Workouts 112

General Guidelines for Exercising During Pregnancy 112
    Lower Body Strength Training During Pregnancy 113
    Home Gym Equipment Basics for the Expectant Mother 113

54. Downward Facing Dog 115

55. Side Leg Lifts with Shoulder Press 116

56. Squats to Side Leg Lifts with One Arm Lateral/Front Raises 117
    How to Stop Night Leg Cramps 118

57. Floor Leg Lifts 119

58. Resistance Band Side Twists 120

59. Standing Glutes Back Kicks. 122

60. Lateral Walks 123

61. Goblet Squat 124

Index of Exercises 126

Special Bonus 130

References 132

Disclaimer

The information contained in this book in no way constitutes medical advice or therapy. The workout routines provided are designed for people in good health. If you have any concerns about your health or suffer with any other medical conditions, you are strongly advised to consult your doctor before you begin any exercise routine.

If you choose not to obtain the consent of your doctor, the author or publisher cannot accept responsibility for any injury or illness which occurs from using the information offered in this book.

Section One: Introduction

In addition to a sensible diet plan and regular cardio exercise, strength training (or resistance training) is undoubtedly the most effective way of becoming a leaner and firmer.

Why Lower Body Strength Training is Important

The leg, hip and glutes muscles all work in combination with each other. When one is injured, the other is often affected. Any exercises that help strengthen, sculpt, firm and define lower body muscles will above all benefit your legs.

In addition to the spine and the wrist, the hip is one of the most commonly fractured parts when bones lose density. [1]

In fact, one-third of people who'll reach 90 will fracture their hip. [2]. And though the age of 90 is probably an eternity away for most, the decline in bone and muscle mass occurs long before your golden years — as these cheery stats reveal:

- Between the ages of **30 and 35**, both muscle and bone begin to break down. [3]

- Muscle shrinks by about **10%** between the ages of 24 and 50, the biggest drop occurring between 50 and 60 years of age — *30%*. [4]

- Muscle mass and strength is less well maintained in the lower body than the upper. [5]

- Additionally, by your forties or fifties, metabolism slows down. It's estimated that **200 to 300** fewer calories are burnt a day. [6].

Getting your weight training in sooner rather than later (although it's never too late to start) can help slow down this decline.

The Benefits You Gain From Strength Training

Strength training helps build stronger bones and when combined with cardio, it increases stamina [7]. It also improves posture and makes everyday activities, such as lifting and carrying, much easier. However, one of the biggest benefits gained from resistance training is the metabolic boost your body receives (more on this in **section three**).

Rather than excessively bulking you up, as mistakenly thought by some, strength training does quite the opposite. The typical woman who strength trains actually shrinks in body size by losing fat and gaining lean muscles, due in part to the occurrence of **EPOC**. [8].

The EPOC Boost: The Post Exercise Fat Sizzler for Added Weight Loss

A key reason why weight training is so good at promoting fat and weight loss is that it amplifies the naturally occurring activity of **excess post-exercise oxygen consumption (EPOC)**. In plain lingo, this is the number of calories your body burns after a workout session [9] [10].

In essence, the harder your body has to work to reload oxygen stores, repair muscles and expel metabolic waste, the more fat calories you burn — even *after* your exercise session is over [11] [12]. In fact, the effects are known to last for more than 38 hours, [13] all of which is a blessing when trying to slim your lower limbs!

What's in This Book?

In this book, you'll find over **60** moves which target and tone major lower body muscles. They include many variations using dumbbells, resistance bands and bodyweight moves.

For added benefit, we've included lots of compound exercises. Compound moves are extremely successful at slimming you down for a number of key reasons:

- **They allow you to do more in less time [14]**
- **They accelerate fat loss [15]**
- **And as noted, they make those everyday movements we take for granted much easier to do**

Contained in this book are fully illustrated step by step exercises ranging from beginner to advance. They can be used to build your own exercise routine, and even better, take around a minute or less to do! What's more, you'll find tips, easy guidelines and other useful nuggets to help you get the most out of your routines.

As a final important note, if you have any concerns about your health or suffer with back problems, you should speak with a doctor before you begin any exercise routine. Furthermore, if you experience any strain or pain during exercise, stop immediately. Strengthen your muscles first with workouts you're able to do without strain, and then try more challenging moves when you feel ready.

Section Two: Basic Stretching

"Blessed are the flexible, for they shall not be bent out of shape." - Coach Kris, nanduryland.com

Stretching exercises are probably one of the most overlooked routines when it comes to fitness.

They are an important part of any exercise workout because they help stretch and limber up your muscles, and increase both respiration and body temperature.

Ideally, stretching should be done for several minutes and can include raising and stretching the arms, bending the knees, touching the toes, twisting the torso and some light cardio. Stretching can be done to 'wake up' the body in the morning or to unwind after a workout or a hectic day.

Creating Your Own Basic Stretching Routine

You can come up with a ritual of your own which the body can become accustom to.

To develop a tailored routine of your own, try out an exercise over a period of time. You can then pick the ones you feel most comfortable with and believe you need most.

Never push any movement or stretch as you may injure yourself.

Ankle Flex

Targets: Ankle Joint, toe extenders

Standing hip width apart, extend one leg in front. Flex your ankle, pulling top of big toe towards you. Hold for 10 seconds. Relax back to centre and then flex your ankle, pointing big toe downwards. Return foot to floor to complete one rep. Repeat 5-10 times and then perform stretch with the opposite leg.

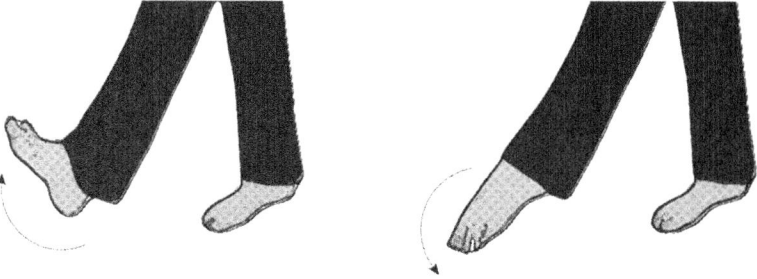

Repeat the same flexing action, but this time, point big toe of foot from side to side (as shown).

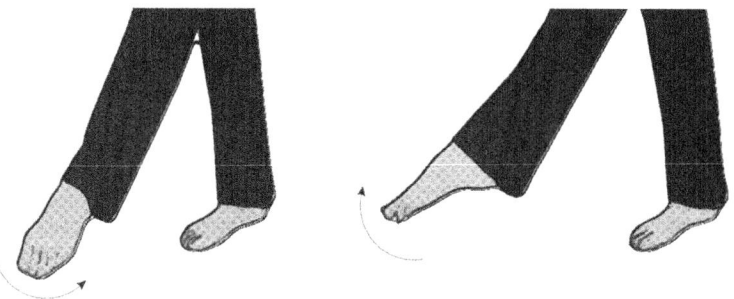

For this exercise, you can place hand on a wall or chair for support, or perform the exercise sitting down.

Toe Balances

Targets: Core and calves

Stand with feet together, resting hands on hips. While slowly lifting heels and rising on toes, engage core, raise arms in front at shoulder level, palms facing downwards. Hold for 15 seconds, and then slowly lower arms and heels back down to ground. Repeat exercise 5 times in total.

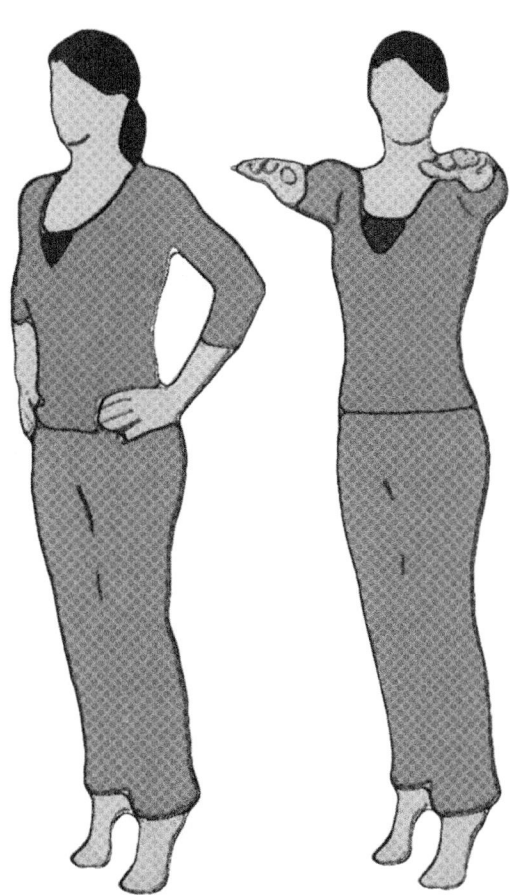

Standing Calf Stretches

Supported:

Facing a wall or chair, step a few inches away from it.

Move one foot back shoulder width distance, keeping it straight with foot flat on floor.

As you bend other leg, lean forward and place hands on the wall. Keep on leaning forward (making sure back foot remains flat on floor) until you feel a stretch at calf. Hold 30 seconds.

This is one rep. Repeat 2 more times, and then switch sides.

Unsupported:

Begin by placing hands on hips and then repeat the steps as described above.

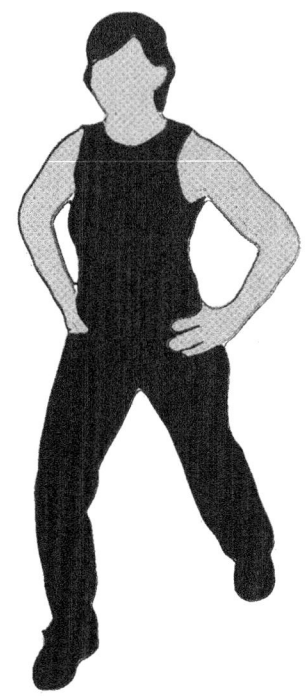

Quad Stretch

Start move by assuming lunge position down on floor, with one leg forward and bent at a 90 degree angle to floor.

Keeping other leg straight, stretch out through heel (as if you are putting that heel on the floor). With hips facing front, simultaneously press pelvis down and lift thigh of your straight leg upwards.

The stretching action of this exercise should be the pelvis pushing down and the thigh pulling up.

Hold for 30 seconds, and then repeat stretch again on same side. Switch legs and perform for 2 repetitions.

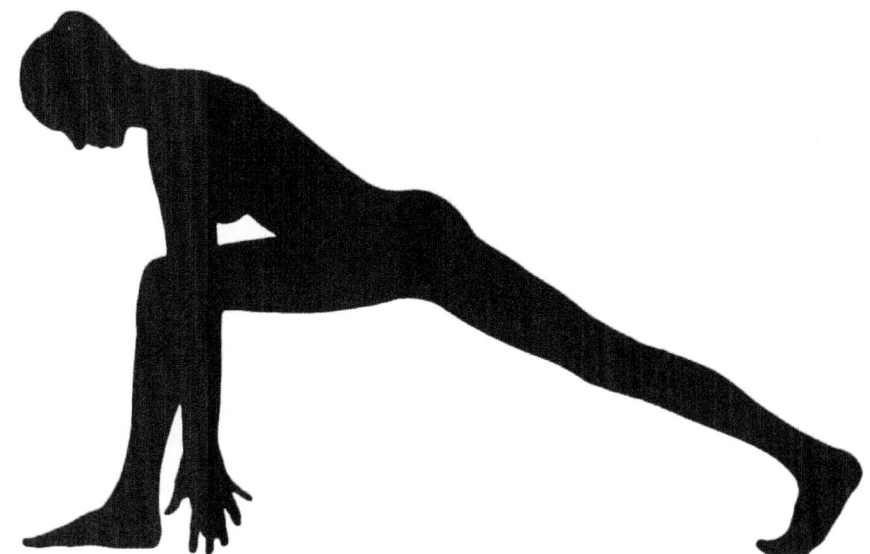

Inner Thigh Stretch

Lie on floor near wall with shoulder towards wall, and then swing legs up wall. Place enough distance between you and wall, so you can straighten legs and completely support lower back.

Slowly widen legs as far as they'll go to sides, allowing gravity to pull legs open until you feel stretch along inner thighs.

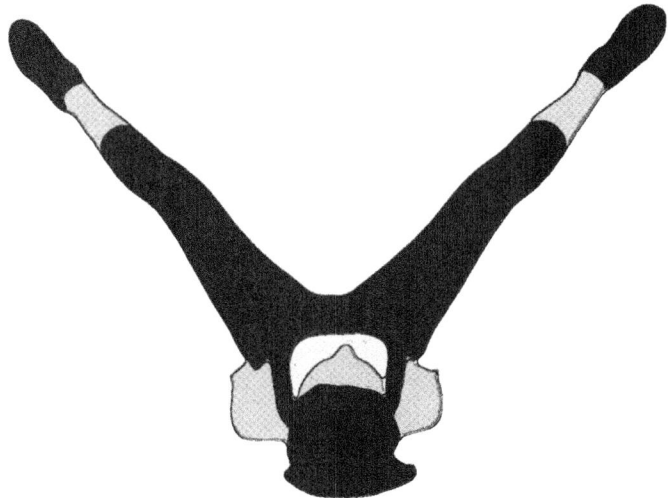

Remain in pose for 30-60 seconds. End move by bending knees, drawing them towards chest. Roll onto side.

For comfort, place a small towel or pillow under head.

Lying Piriformis Stretch (for Rotator Muscles)

Start by lying on back with knees bent and feet flat on floor. Next, cross one leg over other, holding hands behind bottom leg.

Pull both legs towards chest and hold for 30 seconds. You should feel stretch in gluteals muscles of crossed leg. Relax for a moment and then repeat move once more before switching legs.

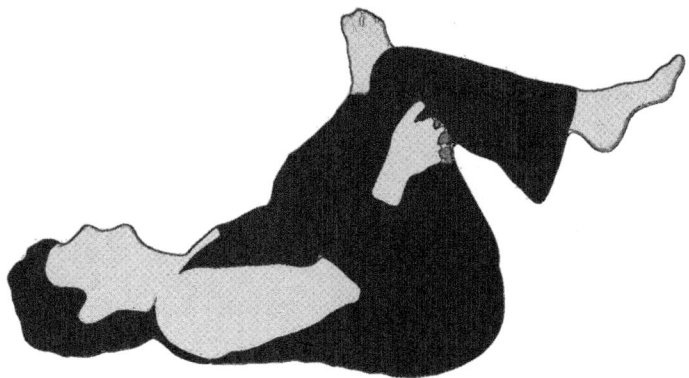

Standing Hamstring Stretch

Targets: Hamstring muscle group

Stand up straight in front of fitness ball (or a low chair or stool). Place one leg on top of ball and hands on hips.

Without rounding lower back, lean forward from hips until you feel a stretch. Hold for 30 seconds and then release stretch. Repeat on the other side.

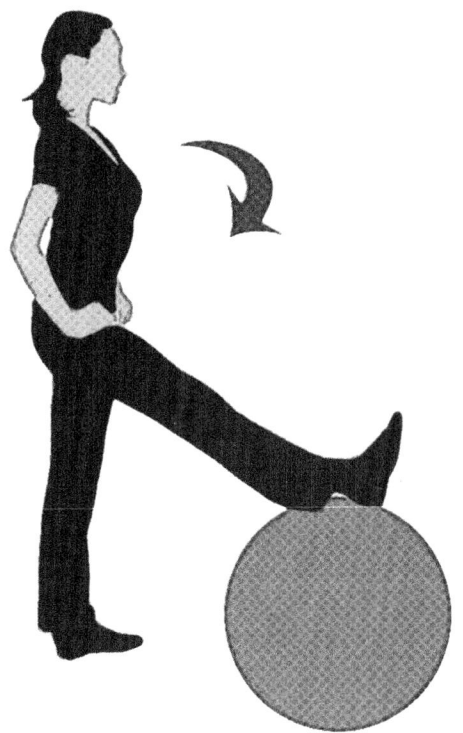

Shin and Ankle Stretches

Targets: Ankle Joint, toe extenders and shin

Begin by kneeling with shins flat on ground, backside seated over both heels and feet extend back.

Gradually lean back and place arms either side with fingers pointing inwards (as pictured). Slowly increase pressure until you feel stretch. Hold and then return to start.

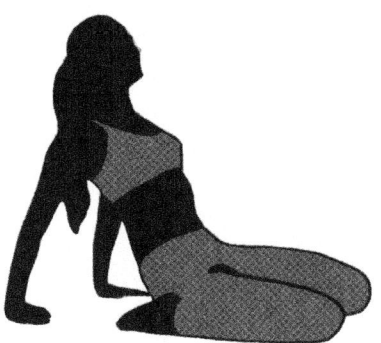

Standing Full Body Stretch

Targets: Abs, back, legs and arms

Begin by standing with feet close together. Slowly raise heels off floor and extend hands above head towards ceiling.

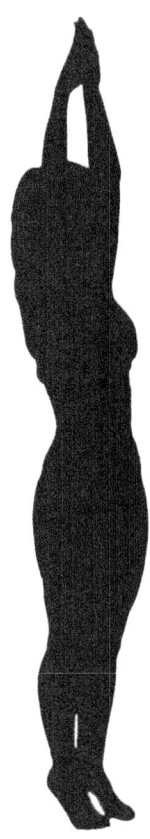

Stretch by pulling upwards throughout entire body. Hold for 30 seconds and then release.

Lean Legs Tip:

Learn How to Stretch in 3 Moves

There are several types of stretching moves, 3 of which are dynamic, static and myofascial [16].

When combined in a planned and simple way, you can help train your muscles to expand and contract rapidly for flexibility, as well as promote healing between workouts.

Dynamic stretching: Moving your arms and legs through a variety of movements without stopping to hold any position. Best to do before your exercise and after a light cardio warm up. For these types of stretches, keep the motion smooth and controlled [17].

Dynamic Stretching Examples: lunges, shoulder circles, arm swings and side bends

Static stretching: Stretching a muscle as far back as you can without pain and then holding it there. Best to do after your workout. Hold each stretch for 30 seconds [18].

Static Stretching Examples: shoulder, chest and upper back stretches.

Myofascial stretching: Applying pressure to different muscles by sliding parts of the body over a foam roller, and these stretches can be done at any time. Press as much of your body weight into the foam roller as you can. Spend 1-2 minutes per myofascial technique [19].

Myofascial Stretching Examples: hamstring myofascial, upper back myofascial and quads myofascial [20]

Back Stretch on Fitness Ball

Start by sitting on ball. Lean back slowly and walk feet out, positioning ball under spine.

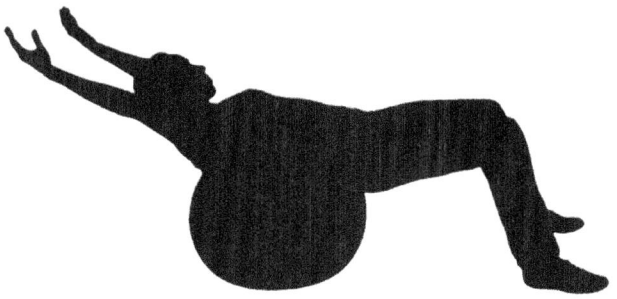

Walk feet away from you to straighten legs. Reach arms up overhead and begin relaxing hips

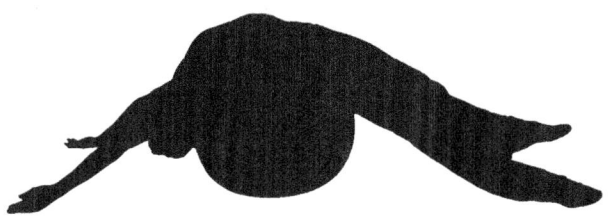

Stretch through core and let arms relax to sides. Hold for 30-60 seconds, breathing deeply throughout. Walk yourself back to start.

Lying Leg Extensions

Targets: Back of thighs

Start by lying flat on floor, knees bended with feet flat on ground.

Raise and extend one leg straight up and hold with both hands around knee or calf.

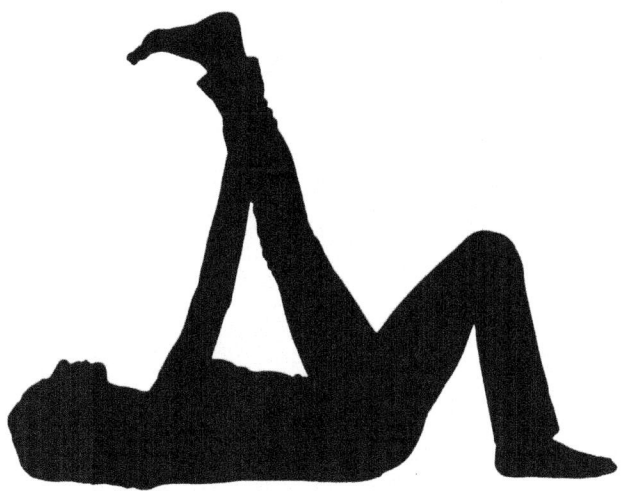

As you breathe slowly and deeply, pull leg closer towards you until you feel a comfortable stretch. Hold for 30 seconds. Release and lower leg. Repeat move with other leg.

Power Skips

Targets: hip, glutes, quad and calves

Leading with one leg, skip as high as possible, raising knee towards chest, while simultaneously driving opposite arm upwards overhead (for momentum).

Keep other leg straight and other arm slightly bent at side. Gently land on foot, and then repeat move with opposite arm and leg. Do move for 15-30 seconds.

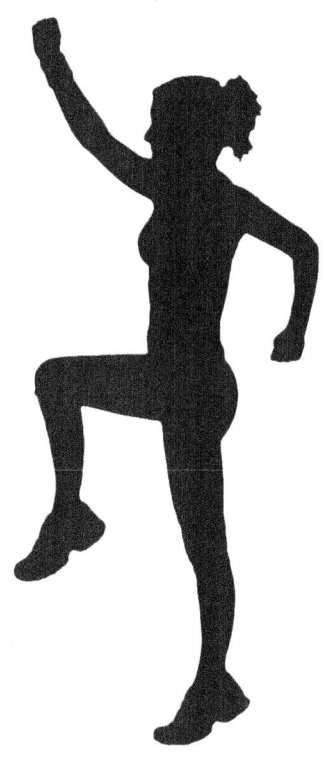

Hip Swings

Targets: Hip joints and adductors

Laying one side with one hip on top of other, use elbow to support yourself up. Lift top leg to hip height and point toe out to side.

In a controlled manner, swing leg out to front as far as possible, keeping torso still. Swing leg in opposite direction, making sure that you don't wobble or jerk as you swing backwards.

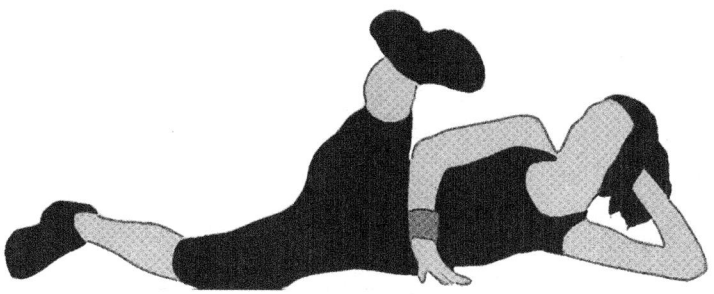

Repeat exercise for 30 seconds and then switch sides.

Straight Leg Kicks

Targets: Quads, hips and butt

Stand normally and extend one arm out straight in front of you parallel to floor.

As you begin walking forwards at a slow pace, kick one leg up as high as you can, aiming foot towards corresponding hand. Kick other leg up, again aiming foot towards corresponding hand.

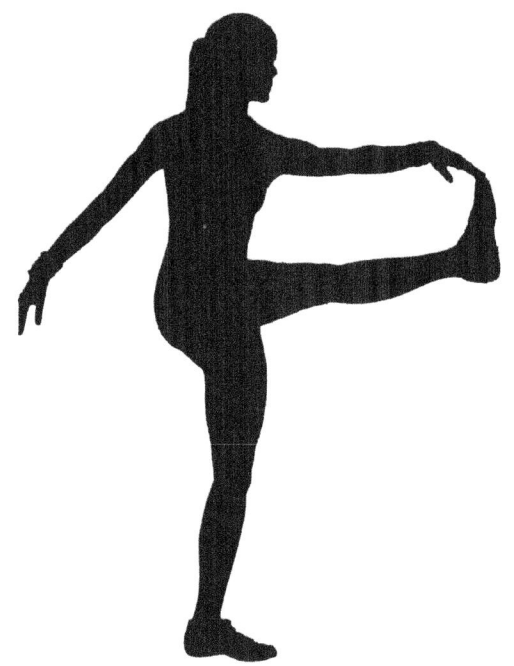

As you do kicks, keep both back and legs as straight as possible. Repeat exercise for 30 seconds.

High Knees

Targets: Quads, calves, glutes

Using a pushing movement, begin jogging in place, raising one knee and opposite arm into air as high as you can.

As you lower back to start, swiftly push other knee and arm up as once before. Continue jogging movement on spot for 30 seconds. Make sure you that your back doesn't arch as you perform exercise.

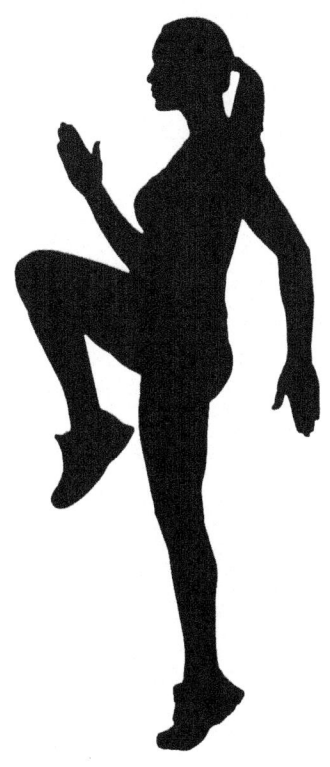

Marching on the Spot

As before, use a pushing momentum to get started, however this time, march on spot.

Raise one knee and opposite arm to hip height, while driving arms up and down in pace with steps. Keep back straight and elbows bent throughout.

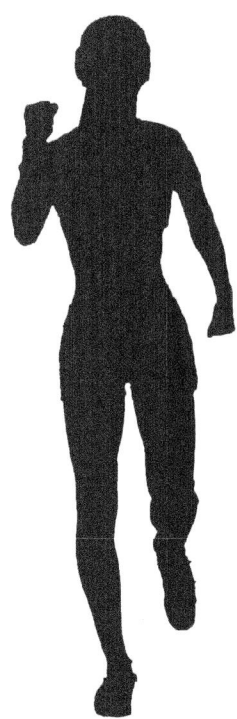

Continue to march in place for one 30 second rep. Repeat for another 30 second rep if desired.

Section Three: Beginners Workouts

You'd be glad to know that it's never too late (or hard) to work your way to toned and slimmer legs, nor does it require the use swanky fitness widgets — just some resistance and enough space to exercise.

As noted in our introduction, not only will you tone up, you'll also build lean muscle. And though the words 'build muscle' spooks out some women, more muscle equals a higher metabolic resting rate [21]. This means that once muscle is stimulated, you'll be burning calories with everything that you do — even for hours after your workout (aka, the EPOC boost) [22].

And if the idea of developing leaner muscles still makes you feel a little nervous, know that muscle is **metabolically active tissue**, which is a fancy way of saying that it's burning fat.

Fat, in contrast, hoards calories and provides insulation, which is all well and good, but when it piles up, it sits around putting stress on your back, joints and heart.

The important point here is that by doing weight training just 3 times a week [23], you'll gain a lot more strength, feel a great deal nimbler on your toes, and have a lot less jiggle to be annoyed about! Enough said.

Basic Lower Body Exercise Guidelines for Beginners

The following basic guidelines are based on advice from **Weight Training For Dummies**, by Georgia Rickard, Liz Neporent, Suzanne Schlosberg [24-28]:

- Begin exercising the bigger muscle groups prior to the smaller ones in this suggested sequence: **glutes, quads, hamstrings, inner and outer thighs, calves, and shins**.

- Perform at least 4 or 5 lower body exercises regularly.

- Your routine should include **compound exercises** — involving several muscle groups at once — and **isolation exercises** — targeting one muscle group.

- If you have weak knees or hips, concentrate on exercising the muscles around those joints for a few weeks, *before* moving on to compound routines. For specific low impact exercises, **please see section nine in this book**.

- **You will ache!** You'll probably experience soreness a couple days after your first few leg exercises. If using dumbbells, to minimize soreness, start with light weights.

Some General Workout Tips

Keep it simple: some of the best legs exercises are the basic ones. These include squats, lunges, leg extensions and many more included in this book.

Always warm up before doing your reps: as noted in our opening section, warming up gets your muscles limber, increases your circulation, improves your flexibility and more importantly, minimizes sprains and tears.

Always use proper form: properly executed routines can yield just as good or even better results than machine workouts. Conversely, bad or sloppy form can lead to injury. Keeping your reps short allows you to maintain your focus and keeps your moves more precise and effective.

Be patient and persistent: don't beat yourself up about your progress. With a *consistent* routine containing some basic moves, you can see incredible results in less than 30 days!

To expedite strengthening and toning of lower limbs, you should add some form of aerobic exercise to your strength training routine, such as swimming, stair climbing, biking or walking.

In this section, you'll find a number of simple, 'living room friendly' exercises for beginners, targeting quads, hamstrings, thighs, glutes and calves.

1. One Leg Balance

Targets: Core, glutes, inner thighs

Standing hip width apart, extend arms outwards to each side. Lift one leg off floor, raising knee to hip level (as shown), hold for 30 seconds and then lower. Repeat move with opposite leg. Perform exercise 5 times in total for each leg.

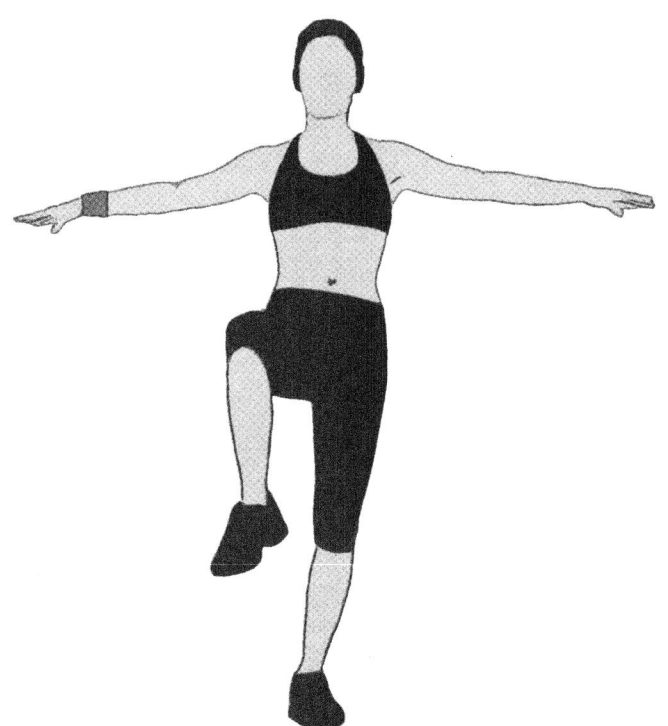

Note: You should feel your hip muscles tightening as you perform this move.

2. Table Top Balance on Fitness Ball

Targets: Core and glutes

Place head, neck and shoulders on fitness ball, knees bent and buttocks on floor.

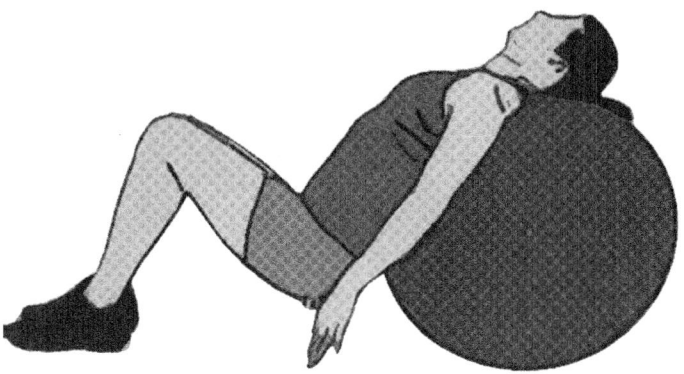

Press heels into ground, lift hips upwards and contract glutes, until body is parallel to floor and knees at 90 degrees.

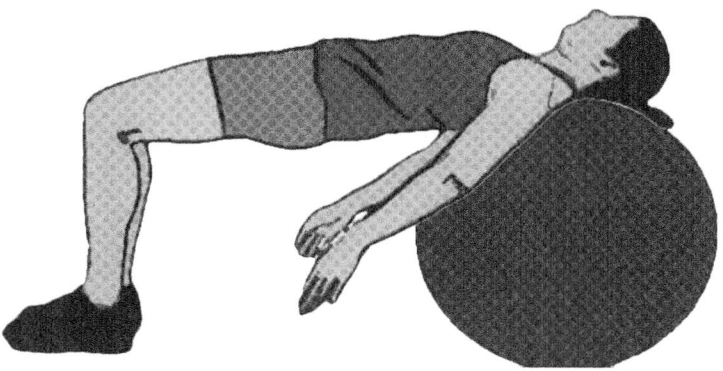

Lower hips and butt back to start. Do 10 reps.

3. Side Step-outs with Knee Raise

Targets: Inner thighs

Stand tall, shoulder width apart and knees slightly relaxed. Move quickly to one side for a second, pause and then lift knee as high as you can towards chest. Lower foot to ground.

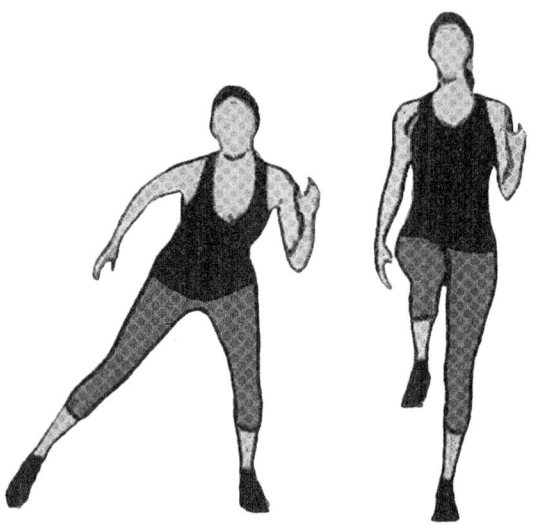

Move quickly to opposite side, lifting other knee to chest, returning foot back to floor. Repeat movement at a steady pace for 60 seconds. Rest for 10 seconds, and then repeat for another 60 second rep.

4. Step-ups with Arm Raises

Targets: Glutes, hamstrings, core

Stand tall with one leg on step bench or bottom step of stairs. Push heel into step, kick other leg out to side and drive arms upwards, keeping core engaged throughout. Step back down to start.

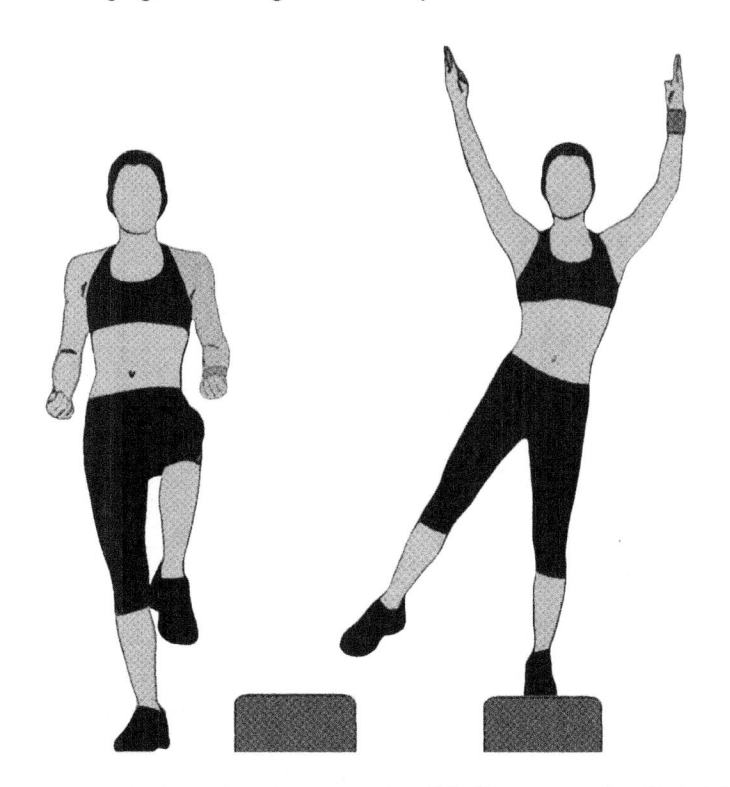

Repeat movement at a steady pace for 30-60 seconds. Rest for 10 seconds, and then repeat move with other leg.

5. Inner Thigh Lifts

Targets: Inner thighs, abs

Laying one side with one hip on top of other, use elbow to support yourself up. Bend top knee and rest leg on floor, with knee parallel with hip.

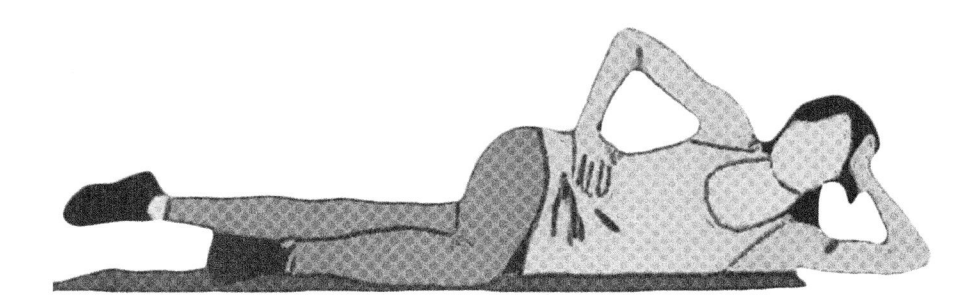

Lift bottom leg as high as you can, pointing toe out to side. Hold for a second, and then slowly lower leg. Repeat for 10 and then turn over and perform same move with other leg.

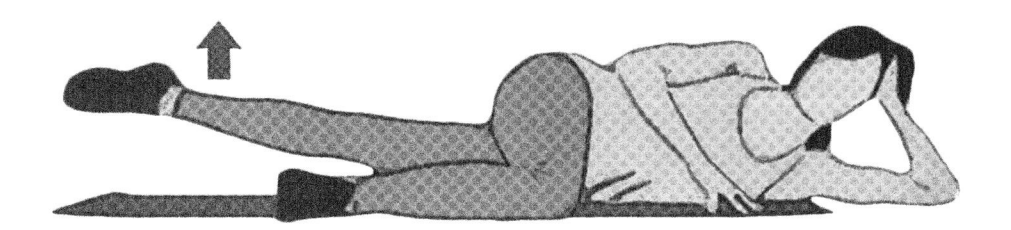

6. Outer Thigh Lifts

Targets: Outer thighs, abs

Begin move in same position, but this time, bend bottom knee, resting leg on floor, with knee parallel with hip (as pictured).

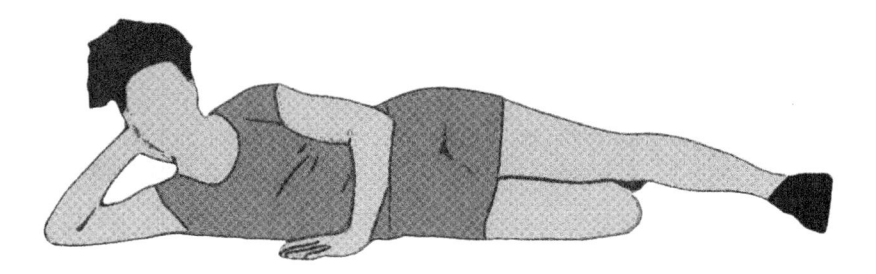

Lift top leg as high as you can, pointing toe out to side. Hold for a second, and then slowly lower leg. Repeat for 10 and then turn over and perform same move with other leg.

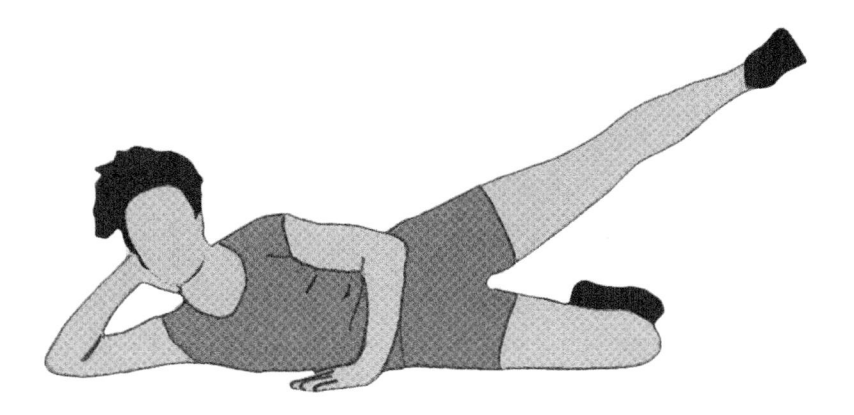

Lean Legs Tip:

Is Spot Reduction Fact or Fiction?

Is there such a thing as spot reduction? Well....yes and no!

If you target the thighs only by doing a bunch of leg lifts, for instance, your chances of slimming down are going to be pretty remote.

Continually exercising just one area doesn't burn fat in that one spot. On the other hand, targeting your entire body with particular strength training moves helps increase metabolism high enough so that your body incinerates fat all day long [29]. This will help burn fat all over your body, including your thighs.

No doubt, lower body fat is hard to shift (and you'll learn about some of those reasons in section four) but it <u>can</u> be burned off. And as noted, the key is to create the lean muscle needed to supercharge your metabolism.

7. Hip Lifts

Targets: Hamstrings and glutes

Lie on back, arms at sides, knees bent and feet flat on floor

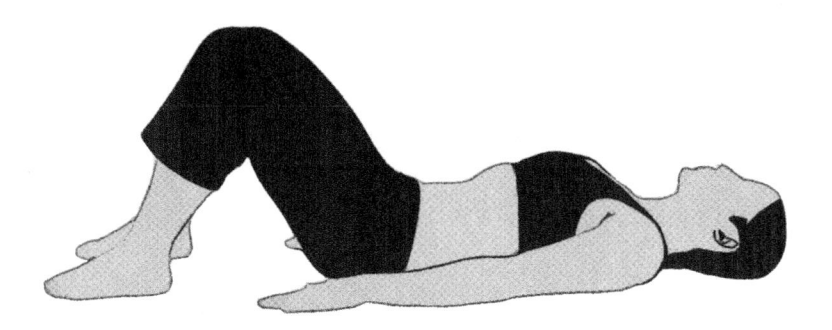

Lift hips upwards. Pause for second, contracting glutes and hamstrings at the top of move, and then lower. Do not overarch spine.

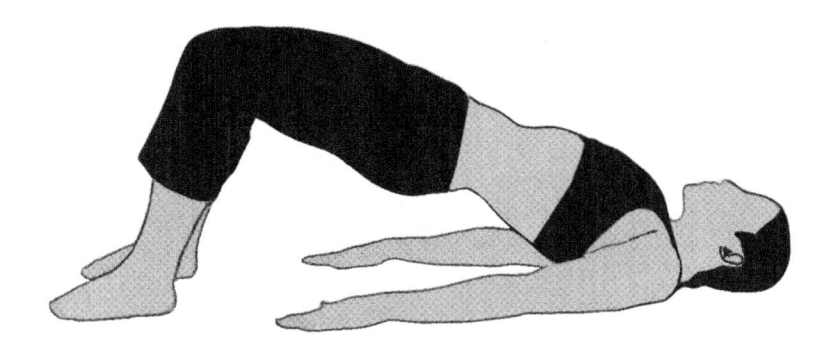

Repeat move for one set of 10 reps. Repeat for another 10 reps if desired.

8. Frog Hops

Targets: Calves, glutes, hamstrings

Start by lowering into shallow squat, feet at hips width distance, arms down by sides, torso upright and head forward.

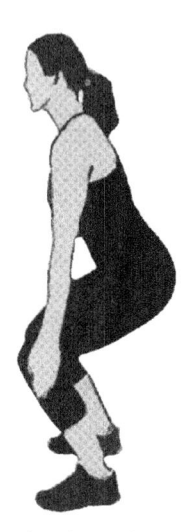

As you jump a few feet forwards, bend arms towards chest, with fists clenched at jaw level. Avoid jumping too high.

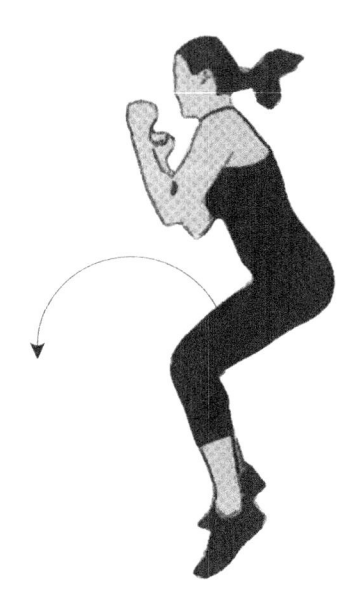

Land with softly bended knees into deep squat on balls of feet, palms flat on floor in front (as pictured) to complete one rep. Repeat move 5 times.

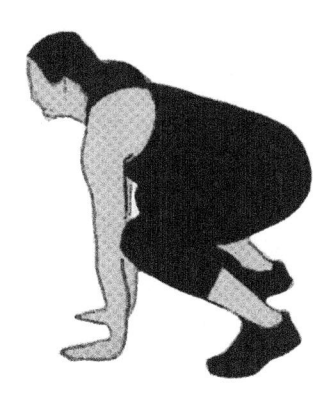

9. Plies

Targets: Glutes, quads, hips, inner thighs, hamstrings, calves

Stand shoulder width apart, knees and toes pointing outwards and hands resting on hips.

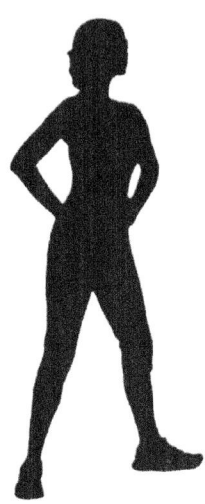

Bend knees and lower hips downwards as low as possible. Keep shoulders and hips aligned, back straight, and knees pointing out over toes.

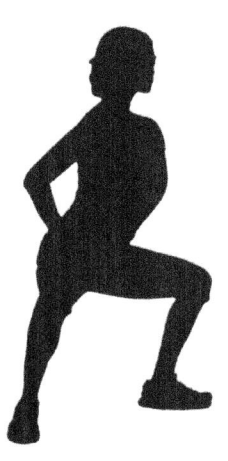

Pause for 10 seconds, and then slowly straighten legs back to start to complete one rep. Perform for 10 reps.

10. Calf Raises

Targets: Calf muscles

Stand with feet close together.

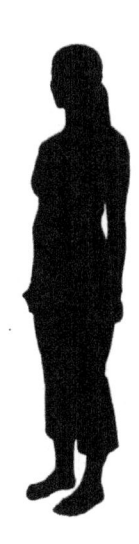

Squeeze calves to lift heels off floor, rising onto balls of feet. Keep back straight and core tight throughout.

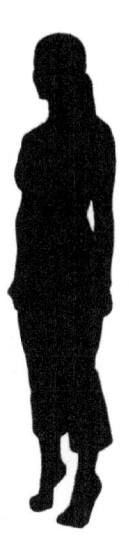

Slower lower, and then repeat move 10 times in total. **This exercise can be performed using a chair for support.**

Section Four: Glutes, Hips and Thighs Workouts

Science has shown that along with our female counterparts in the animal kingdom, women accumulate fat faster and drop pounds far slower [30]. And as luck (and biology) would have it, twice as much fat tends to be stored around a women's hips and thighs than a man's. [31].

The Slow Burn: Why Lower Body Fat is Hard to Shift for Women

Our body fat provides some useful functions. It protects and stockpiles calories in a food crisis, and as nature's designated baby producers, women need the additional fuel to feed junior during pregnancy.

But like stubborn in-laws who can't take a hint, hip and thigh fat comes to stay but simply won't budge, and there are a few reasons why.

Slower Metabolism: Compared to men, women have a lower resting metabolism, and therefore, burn fewer calories to maintain basic life functions (like respiration, digestion, etc). [32].

Hormones: Research has also shown that hip and thigh fat is notoriously difficult shift because that's where hormones choose to store and keep fat. [33]. This is especially so during menstruation.

Estrogen and **progesterone**, which regulate the menstrual cycle, produce somewhat of a 'double whammy' effect on a woman's body.

Estrogen deposits fat in your breasts, hips, glutes, and thighs, by chemically stimulating fat cells in those areas to store fat. On top of that, progesterone chimes in by making you feel hungrier, sleepier, sluggish, and less inclined to exercise [34].

Pregnancy: According to research, women gain about **20%** of body fat from the first trimester until the end of pregnancy [35]. Progesterone levels remain high throughout pregnancy, making you crave more food.

However, the biggest cause of weight gain during pregnancy is fat cells, which are mostly deposited around the upper thighs. [36]

The number of fat cells depends on how much and how fast fat is gained, but once created, fat deposits tend to stick around quite stubbornly, well after the baby is born. [37].

The one exception to this appears to be during breastfeeding. Lactation burns roughly **800 calories a day**, allowing fat on hips and thighs to be burnt to help with milk production in breasts. [38].

3 Tips to Help Your Hips, Glutes and Thighs Win the War Against Biology (and Gravity)

It does seem rather annoying that thighs, hips and glutes are some of the most common places where biology and the law of gravity works against women. But with the right techniques and moves, it is possible to respectfully flip mother nature and Sir Isaac Newton the bird, get slimmer hips and thighs, and restore your backside back to the position it deserves to be.

1: Lunges and squats are your lower body's best friend:
Acknowledged as the ultimate lower body workout by fitness experts, squats work every major part in your lower region — thighs, hips, glutes, shins and calves. It even works the lower back. [39].

One legged squats in particular have been shown to be the best exercise for your glutes. This is because all of your body weight is placed on one foot [40]

As a result, this forces the muscles of just one side to lift your entire body. One legged squats also serve as an excellent balance and strengthening exercise [41].

Like squats, **lunges** also work multiple muscle groups — quads, hamstrings, hip flexors, glutes and calves. Additionally, lunges get you moving in many directions and improve range of motion [42].

2: Use body-weight exercises to tone not bulk: Technically speaking, the lack of testosterone (and other factors) prevents women from amassing the same amount of bulk men do. However, if your desire is to simply get nicely toned legs, you can skip using weights and rely on your body-weight instead.

Lifting your own body weight distributes the exercise load over multiple muscle groups, providing strength and tone without bulk [43].

For leg exercises using body-weight only, see section six of this book.

3: Exercise your glutes often: Your glutes are nothing but muscle — in fact, the most powerful muscles of your entire body. If we don't use them as designed, such as for walking, climbing and so forth, they lose tone and start to droop.

For best results, perform glute workouts **2-3 times a week**, starting with **two sets of 8 to 12 reps**, and work up to **three sets of 10 to 15 reps** for each exercise [44].

Additionally, choose exercises that collectively target gluteals, hamstrings, and the lower-back region for the best all-around toning [45].

In this section you'll find a variety of hip, glutes and thigh exercises that strengthen, tone, and add a cardio element to your workouts.

11. Forward Lunges

Targets: Core, thighs, glutes

Standing hip width apart and with hands on hips, move forward with one leg and slowly lower body, until knee is bent at least 90 degrees.

Push up back to start, and then repeat move with other leg to complete the rep. Perform for 30 seconds, rest for 10 seconds and repeat exercise.

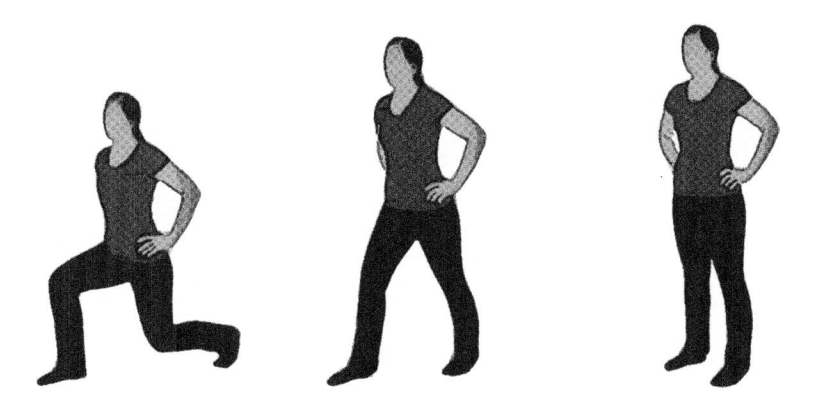

Lean Legs Tip:

Why Forward Lunges Are Great For Glutes and Thighs

Properly and regularly performed lunges are excellent for shaping and toning thighs and glutes. Lunges fire the large muscles groups into action, meaning you'll be burning plenty of energy while doing them [46] — and why they're cited as one of the best exercises for shedding fat [47].

Lunges strengthen muscles that help protect the knees from injury (more on that in **section eight**) promote good movement patterns, and improve balance [48].

Some tips for performing the forward lunge:

- Breathe in as you lower into the lunge and breathe out as you return to start.

- Keep your back upright and straight throughout, and keep working towards maintaining your balance.

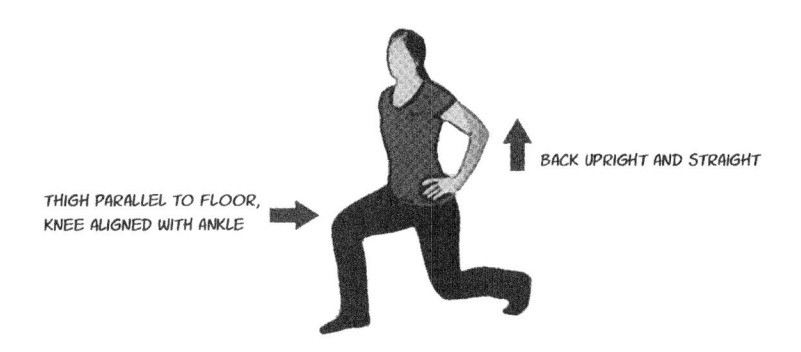

THIGH PARALLEL TO FLOOR, KNEE ALIGNED WITH ANKLE

BACK UPRIGHT AND STRAIGHT

If you feel pain doing this exercise, stop immediately.

For beginners: place hand on a wall or sturdy object to keep steady as you learn the movement.

12. Side Kick Squats

Targets Glutes, quads, inner thighs, hamstrings, calves, core

Begin standing slightly wider than shoulder width apart, toes pointing forward. Lower into squat, elbows bent and fists in front of chest.

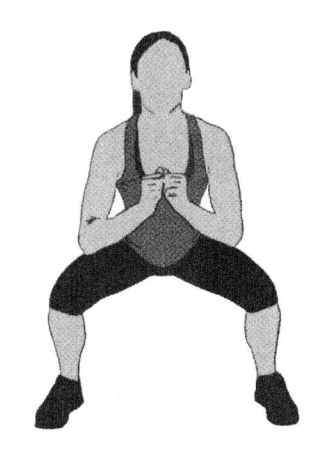

Stand up, lift one leg off floor and kick one leg out to side (as pictured).

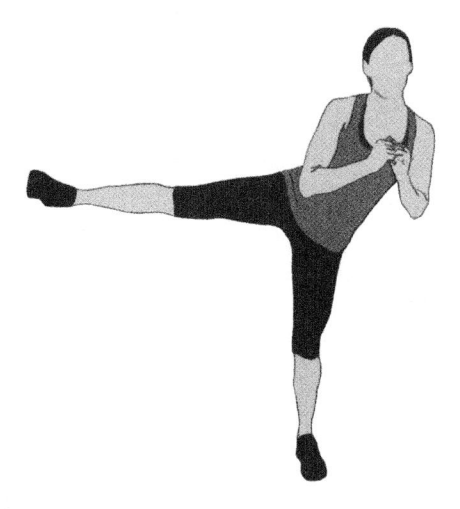

Lower leg back to floor and return to squat to complete rep. Do 10 reps, and then repeat move with other leg.

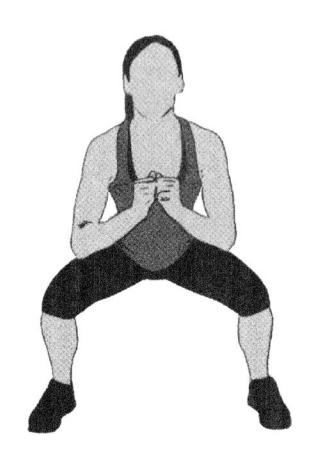

13. Knee thrust to Front Kick

Targets: Hip flexors, glutes

Lead with one foot, knees slightly bent, fists in front of chin, palms facing inwards.

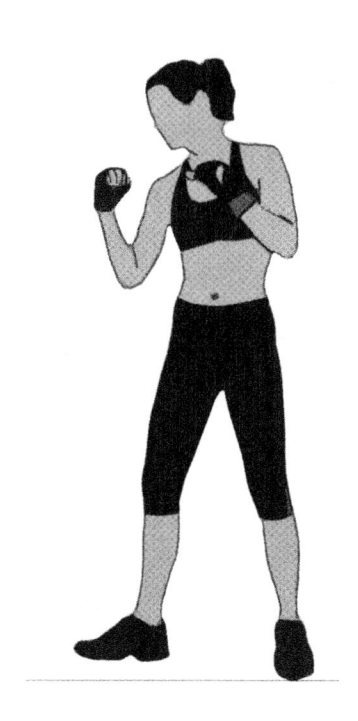

Rotate hips, lift and bend knee of other leg in towards chest.

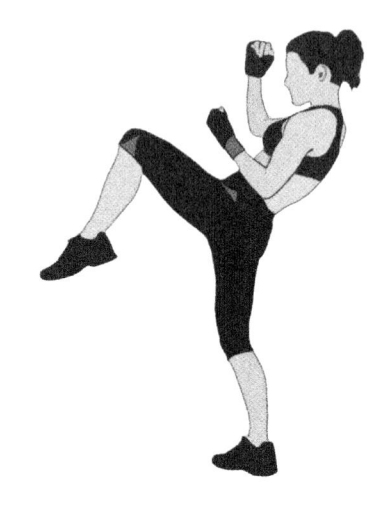

Extend leg in front, leaning slightly back as you push out through heel, foot flexed. Quickly bend knee back in and step down.

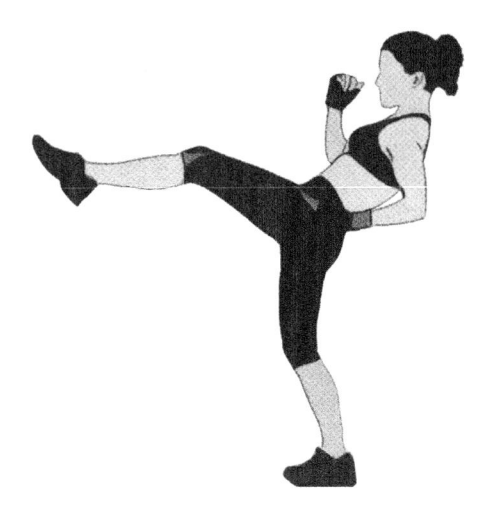

Repeat move 5 times and then switch legs.

14. Side Kicks

Targets: Hip flexors, glutes

Lead with one foot and fists up.

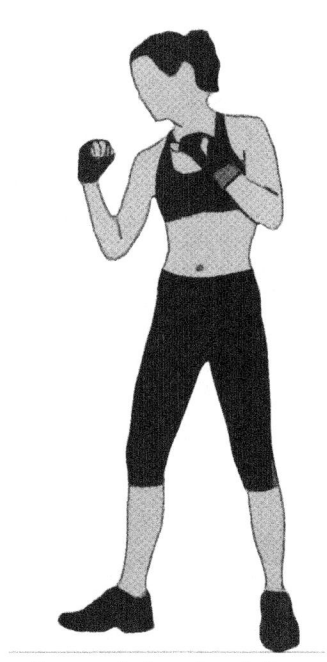

Kick leg to side, pushing through heel, while punching with corresponding arm.

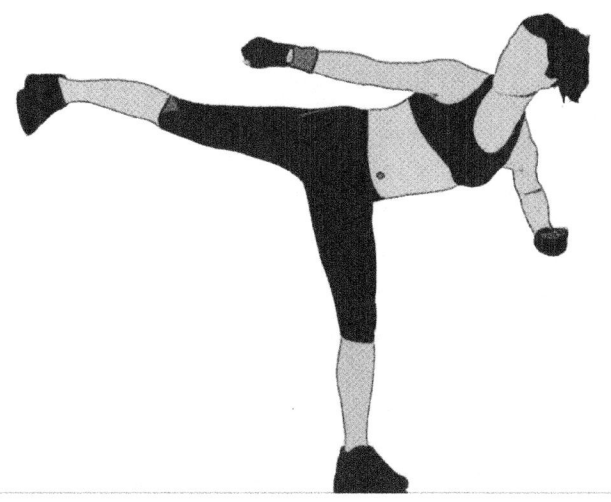

Perform for 10 reps, switching sides with each rep.

15. Kickbacks

Targets: Hamstrings, glutes

Get down on all fours, extend arms in front, palms on floor, back straight and head in line with back.

Keeping back straight and leg bent, slowly lift one foot upwards until thigh is parallel to floor. Hold for a second, and then return start. Perform for 10 reps, and then repeat with other leg.

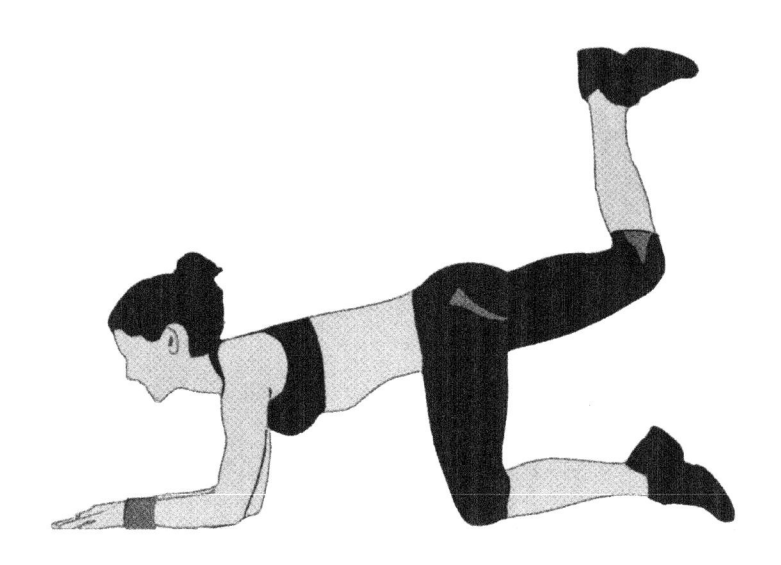

16. Kickbacks with Resistance Band

Targets: Hamstrings, glutes

Begin exercise in same starting position as before, holding ends of a resistance band, wrapping middle of band around bottom of one foot.

Using glute muscles, push one leg back straight, making sure there's tension on band.

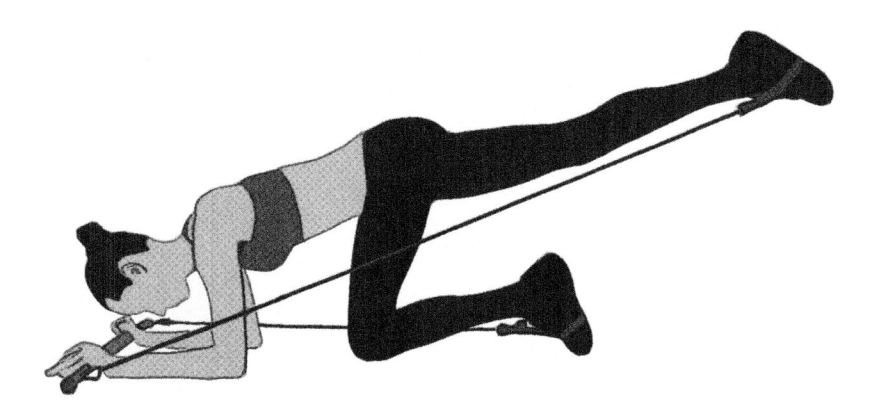

Keep back flat. Hold for a second, and then return to start. Perform for 10 reps, and then repeat with other leg.

17. One Legged Squats

Targets: Hamstrings, hips, quads, glutes, calves

Lift one leg so that you're standing on one leg.

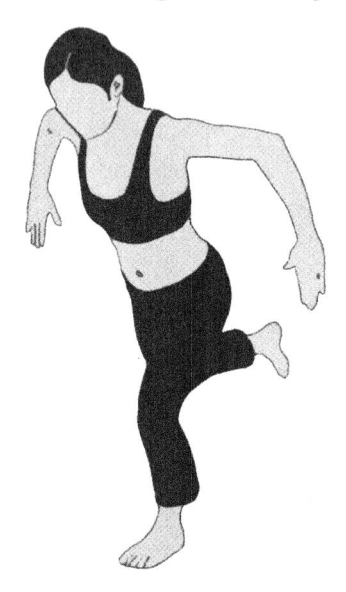

Squat down and lean slightly forward so that thigh is at a slight angle to floor.

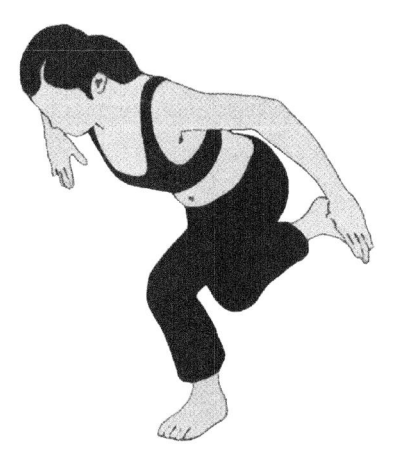

Push back up to starting position to complete rep. Do two sets of 5 reps per leg.

18. Shoulder Width Squats

Targets: Glutes, quads, inner thighs, hamstrings, calves

Standing hips width distance, raise arms in front to shoulder level. Bend knees, keeping back and arms straight, until thighs are almost parallel to floor. Press heels into floor and stand halfway up. Lower again, and then repeat. Do 10 reps in total.

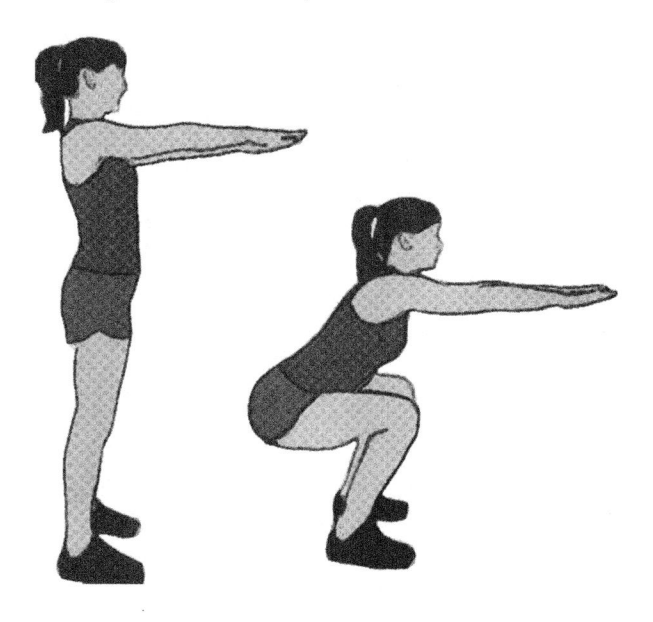

Harder: **Speed Squats** - Assume same starting position as before, but this time repeat squat movements at a faster pace. Perform a 30-60 second rep, resting for 10 seconds, then perform another rep.

19. Dead Lifts

Targets: Shoulders, glutes, core, forearms

Place pair of dumbbells on floor in front. Keep chest up, bend at hips and knees, and then grab dumbbells with overhand grip.

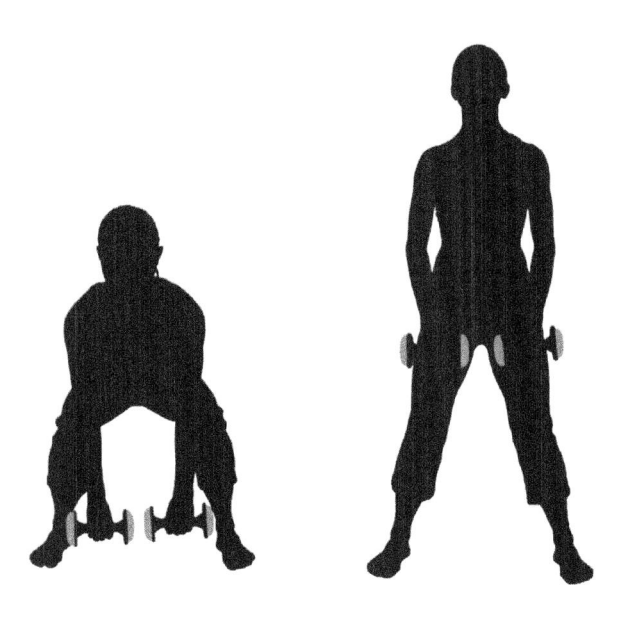

With arms straight and lower back slightly arched (not rounded), push up with legs and feet, forcing hips forwards, pulling upper body back and up.

Slowly lower dumbbells to floor to complete one rep. Do one set of 8-10 reps.

Section Five: Fitness Ball Workouts

If you have a hectic lifestyle or have nil interest in lengthy exercise routines, then the fitness ball may be your best chum.

More Toning Power in Less Time: Why You Get Faster Results Using a Fitness Ball

Fitness or stability balls are considered to be one of the best pieces of exercise equipment for multi-tasking, because they allow you to simultaneously work multiple muscle groups. To all intents and purposes, the fitness ball lets you do more stuff in less time.

You'll also be challenged. When exercising on the ball, you're using muscles through your entire body to stay balanced. In particular, your core [49].

In most cases, a fitness ball routinely places a greater demand on your core muscles than the same exercises without a ball. Even if you're performing an exercise targeting your lower body muscles, such as side leg raises, your core muscles still need to support your upper body [50].

This is much more challenging than doing the same exercise on the floor because you're not only engaging your thighs, hips and glutes, but also your abs, waist and back. In effect, a full body workout.

Additionally, your core muscles have to support your upper body to maintain good posture and create good muscle coordination as you perform the exercise [51].

Research has also shown that when compared to the floor, chair or a weight bench as a workout aid, the fitness ball is more successful at toning you up and slimming you down. [52].

How to Pick the Best Fitness Ball for Your Home Workouts

Generally, a 22-inch (55 cm) fitness ball will suit most people. If you're 5 foot or less, an 18-inch (45 cm) ball will be best. If you're 5 foot 8 or more, choose a 26-inch (65 cm) ball [43].

Fitness balls are available in many fitness and sport shops (and some department stores) in store and online.

By and large, they're made of anti-burst PVC plastic for pliability. Some brands, however, may contain latex. If you have skin sensitivity, you can get latex free fitness balls. Some examples include **Gaiam** and **Gymnic Plus**.

Though this section contains exercises that typically target the lower body, as illustrated, you'll be recruiting a lot more muscles when performing these moves.

20. Lying Hamstring Curl

Targets: Hamstrings, calves, glutes

Begin by lying flat on back, fitness ball under heels and arms straight out to side for support. Lift hips off ground, keeping weight on shoulder blades and feet.

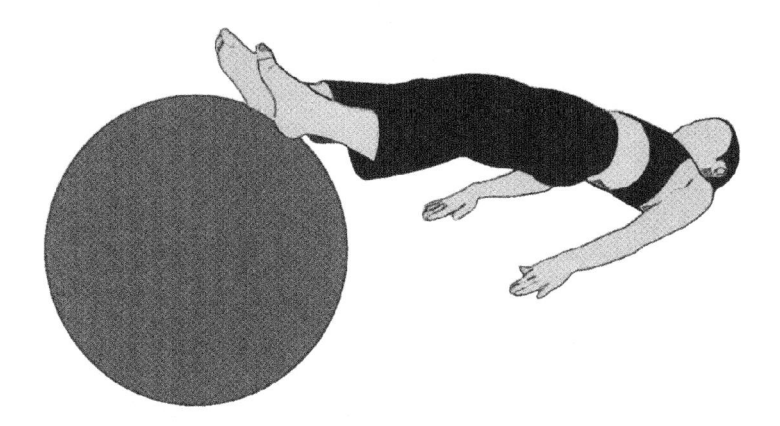

Bend knees and slowly roll ball towards body as you curl heels. Pause briefly, and then return to start with straight legs and hips bridged to finish move. Perform for 10 reps.

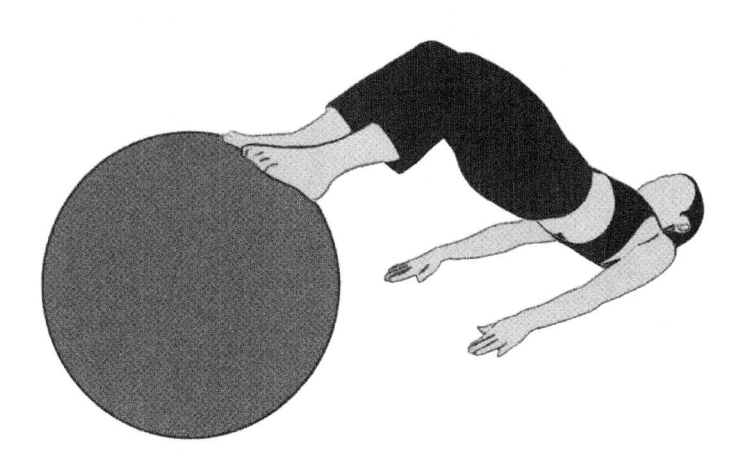

21. Sitting Knee Lifts

Targets: Quads, glutes, hip flexors, core, arms

Sit tall on ball, arms down by sides, legs bent and feet flat on floor at hip width distance.

As you raise one knee, lift opposite arm above head (as pictured). Lower both arm and leg and then repeat movement, raising other leg and opposite arm.

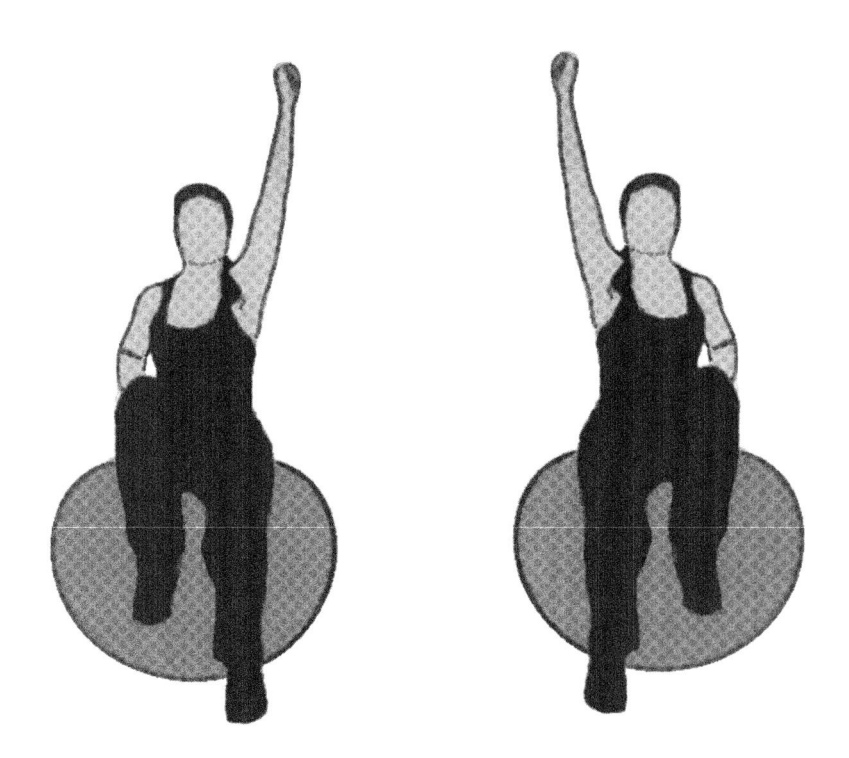

Continue to alternate in this manner at a steady pace for 30-60 seconds. Rest for 10 seconds before repeating another repetition.

22. Standing Knee Lifts

Targets: Quads, glutes, hip flexors, core

Stand with small fitness ball on floor in front.

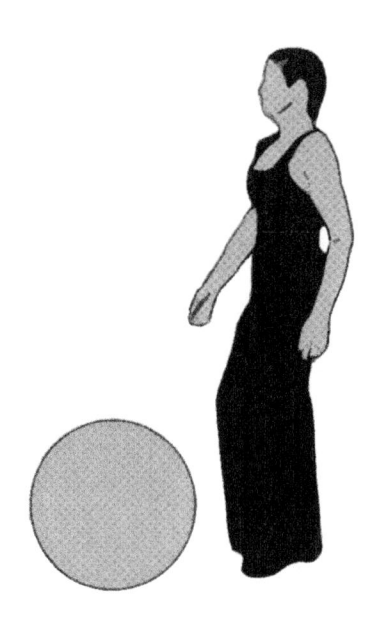

Step to side and as you tap toes of one foot on top of ball, raise opposite arm up to chest level (as pictured).

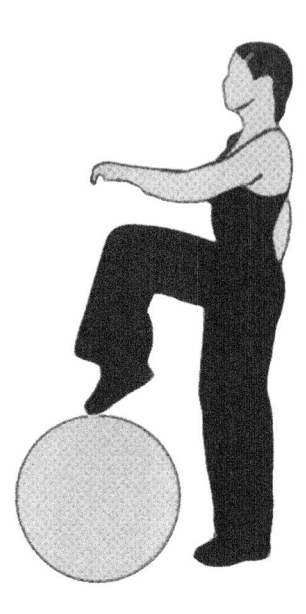

Lower arm and foot to floor. Repeat same movement with opposite arm and leg. Continue to alternate at a steady pace for 30-60 seconds.

Note: As you perform exercise, use arms to drive hips upwards as you tap ball each time.

Lean Legs Tip:

Why Exercise Balls are a Winner for Functional Fitness

Functional fitness trains you to improve strength, ROM and stability so that you may better perform everyday activities, such as bending, twisting, reaching, lifting, etc.

Unlike certain gym machines — which training you to move in one plane — functional fitness tools, such as exercise balls, foam rollers and medicine balls, involve compound exercises, or multi-joint movements that work several muscles or muscle groups at one time.

In this respect, this better prepares you for daily activities, since all of the involved actions require your body to move in a nonlinear, dynamic fashion [54] [55].

Try this functional fitness move on the ball, which targets the back, core and glutes:

Lie face down with chest on top of ball, legs extended behind and feet against wall. Place hands on sides of head.

Breathe in deeply and slowly raise upper body, squeezing shoulder blades as you lift.

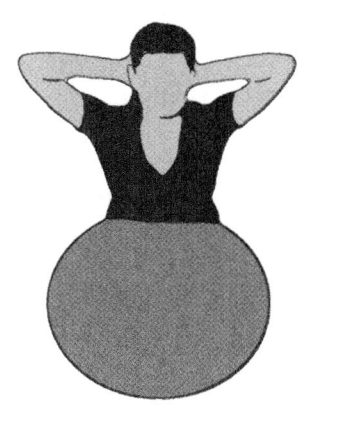

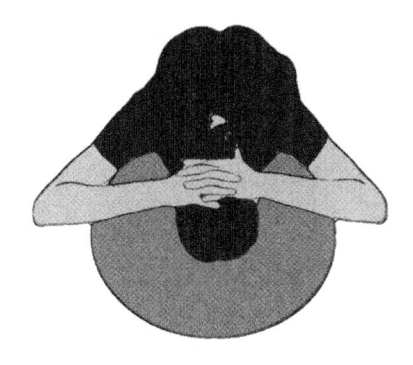

Hold for a few seconds and while breathing out, slowly lower. Perform for 5-10 reps.

23. Bridge

Targets: Core, glutes, hips

Lay on back, knees bent, feet on ball at hip width distance and parallel to one another. Extend arms by side, palms facing downwards.

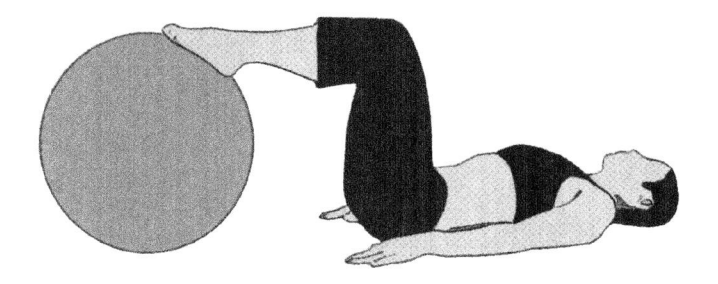

Slowly roll back off floor, pressing feet into ball, bringing body into bridge pose. Hold for 30 seconds, and then slowly bring body back down to ground.

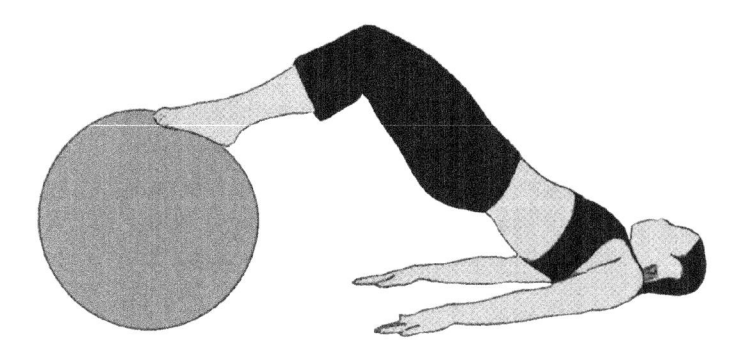

Keep thighs and core strong throughout as you perform move.

24. Standing Leg Swings/Kicks

Targets: Inner and outer thighs, hips

Stand a few inches away from small fitness ball. Place one foot out to side and then using power of hips, swing leg over fitness ball. Repeat movement with opposite leg. Alternate with each leg swing for a total of 10 reps.

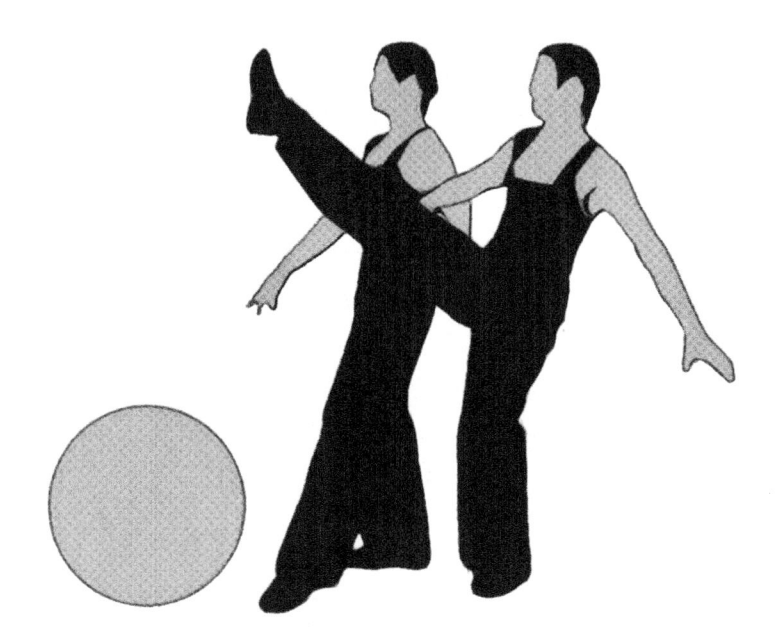

25. Sitting Walks

Targets: Quads, hips, abs

Sit tall on ball, arms down, palms placed on ball, legs bent, and feet flat on floor at hip width distance.

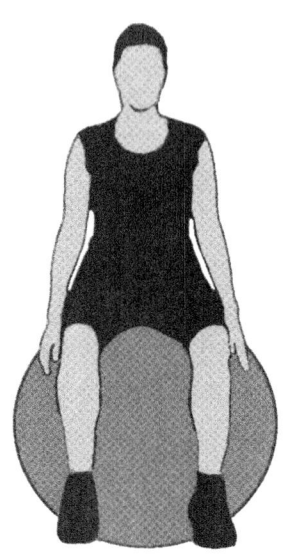

Keep arms in place and raise one knee to chest height. Quickly return foot to floor and then raise other knee.

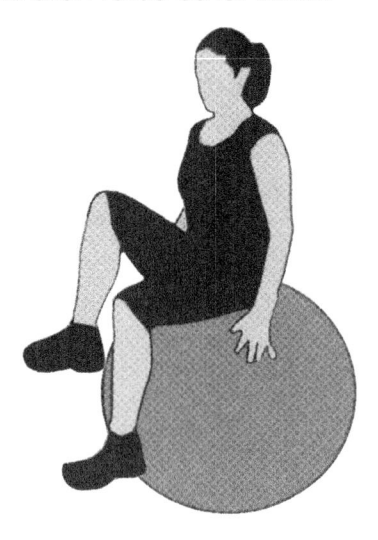

Continue to steadily march or walk on spot for a 60 second rep, keeping back straight throughout exercise.

26. Spilt Squats

Targets: Quad, glutes, hamstrings, abs

Stand upright, arms by sides and with back foot on ball.

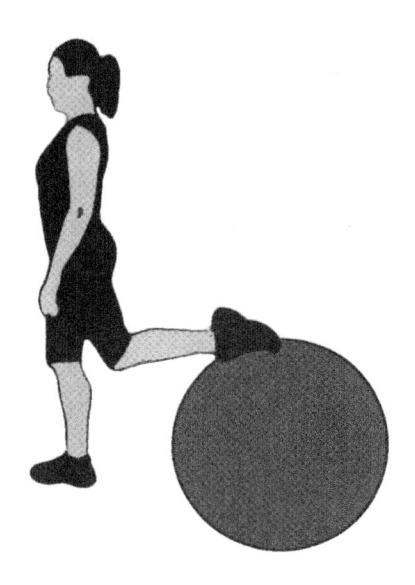

Lower as close to floor as possible. Pause, and then push up. Do 10 reps, switch legs and repeat move.

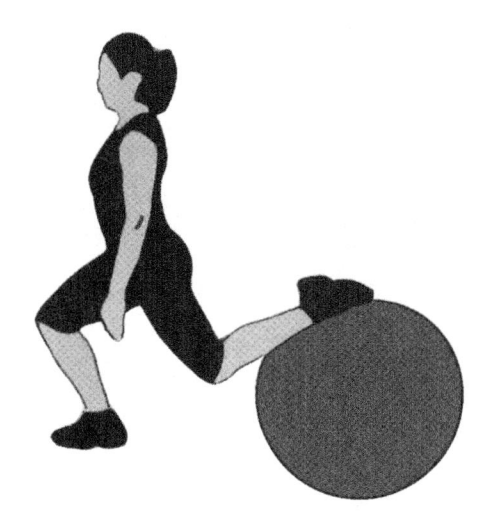

27. Wall Squats

Targets: Quads, glutes, hamstrings, core muscles

Press ball between back and wall.

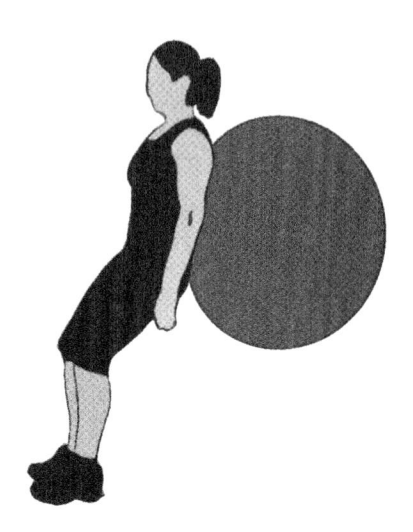

Lower into squat, letting ball roll up back, until upper thighs are parallel to floor. Push down into heels, pause for a second and then rise to complete rep. Do 10 reps in total.

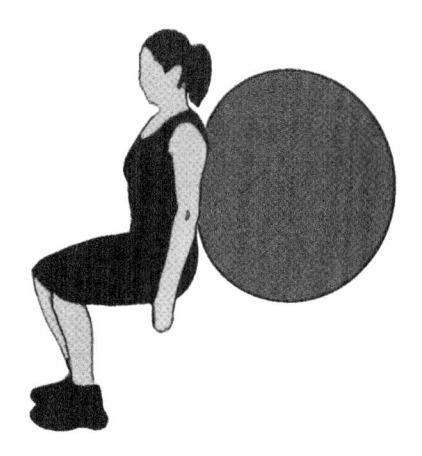

28. Single Leg Wall Squats

Targets: Quads, glutes, hamstrings, core muscles

Begin exercise as before, but this time, lower into squat and when thighs are parallel to floor, lift one leg off ground.

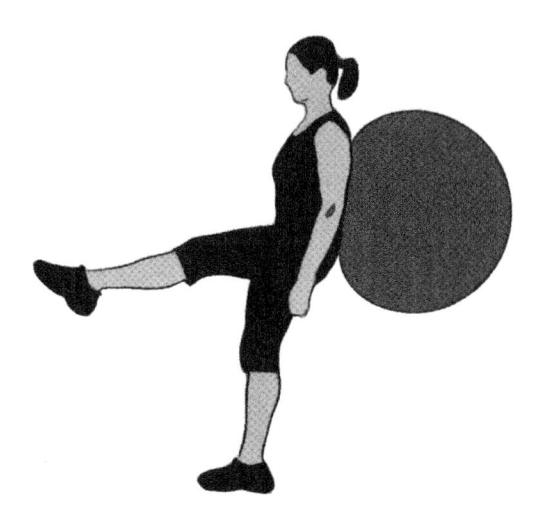

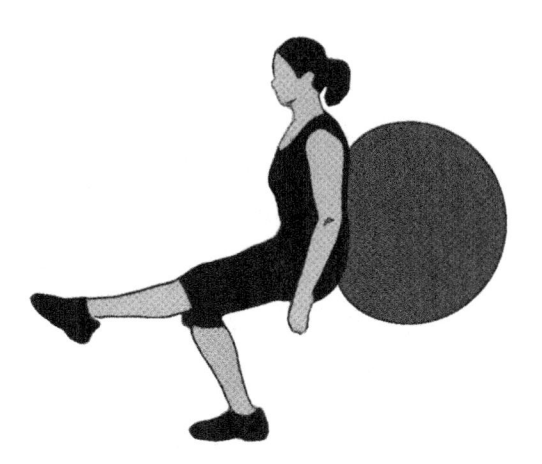

Pause for a second, tighten abs and straighten leg to come to standing position to complete rep. Do 5 reps for each leg.

29. Leg Presses

Targets: Quads, glutes, hamstrings, core muscles

Begin by sitting on ball. Slowly roll down, walking feet forwards until sitting inclined, upper back resting on ball and knees bent (as pictured).

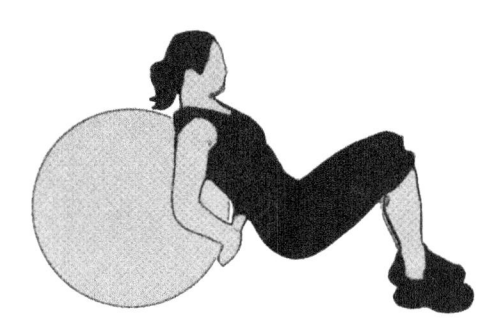

Push through heels of both feet, and then push back on ball until legs are nearly straight. Engage hips and thighs muscles as you perform move. Lower and then repeat for a total of 10 reps.

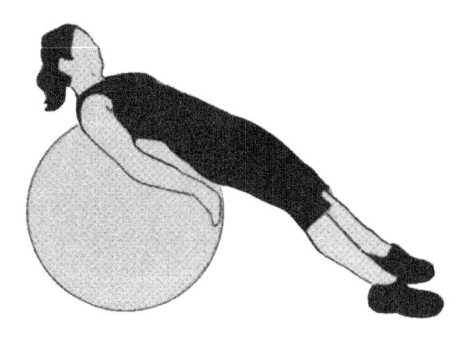

30. Supported Lean Back

Targets: Quads, glutes, hamstrings, abs

Kneel on floor besides ball, knees hip width apart and torso upright. Place one hand on ball and then slowly lean back as far as possible, keeping knees firmly in place.

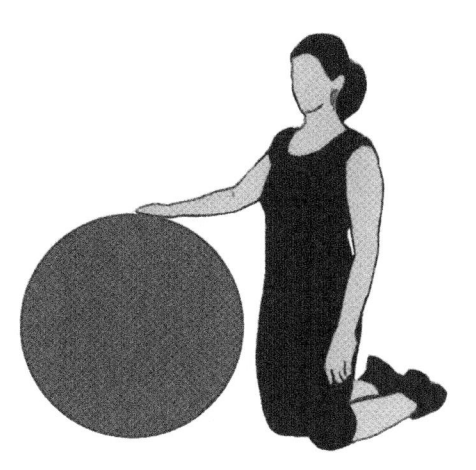

Hold reclined position for a few seconds, and then use core to slowly come back up to start. Do 10 reps.

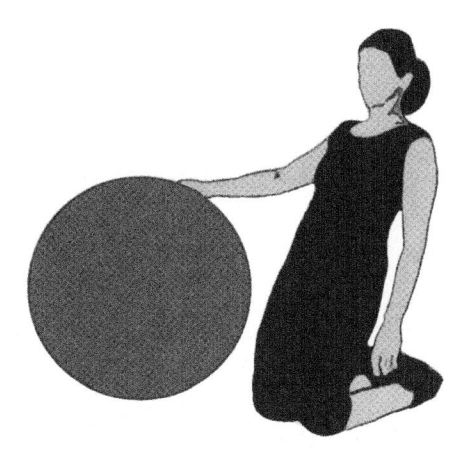

Section Six: Body-weight Workouts

Mark Lauren says you are your own gym, **BJ Gaddour** refers to your body as a barbell, and **Kesh Patel** believes that body-weight training is a key part of development for better health and well-being [56].

However one chooses to view to them, body-weight exercises are one of the best ways for increasing both strength and stamina. They train you to move with better precision — essential to proper exercise form and technique — and can help you work your body without adding lots of equipment.

Benefits of Body-weight Exercises

- **Each movement works multiple muscle groups:** thus making your body work harder which in turn increases metabolism [31].

- Involves simple sequences of movements and normally faster to perform [32].

- Improves strengthen, tone, endurance and stamina [33].

- Can be done in a shorter space of time, performed literally anywhere and at no cost! [34]

Train on One, Rule on Two: Building Stronger Limbs with Single Leg Exercises

Contradictory as it may sound, performing individual exercises on one leg makes you stronger and well balanced in both. Single-legged moves help develop underused muscles, and triggers small supporting muscles around joints [57] [58].

As a result, strength and stability around your ankles, knees and hips are increased [59].

Many of us have one leg that is weaker or not as well developed as the other. Even if you have a strong pair, there is a tendency to slightly favour one leg. This can lead to a disparity that can weaken leg performance, making you more susceptible to injury [60]. Single leg exercises are the most successful approach to redressing these muscle imbalances.

As noted in **section four**, single leg exercises are an excellent way of increasing the weight placed on lower-body muscles — without the use barbells or dumbbells — since each leg is required to hold the mass of your entire body [61].

Finally, single leg training improves postural control, or in layman, controlling your center of gravity over your base of support. This allows your muscles to work more efficiently, so you can move faster [62].

This section contains a simple selection of body-weight moves, however to discover even more examples, good books for further reading are:

"You Are Your Own Gym: The Bible of Bodyweight Exercises" and **"Body by You: The 'You Are Your Own Gym Guide to Total Women's Fitness"**, by Mark Lauren and Joshua Clark, and **"Bodyweight Strength Training Anatomy"**, By Bret Contreras.

31. Jump Squats

Targets: Lower back, abs, glutes, thighs, hamstrings

Stand with feet spread shoulder width apart. Lower into squat, until thighs are parallel to ground. Arch lower back slightly forwards, placing arms downwards in front (as pictured).

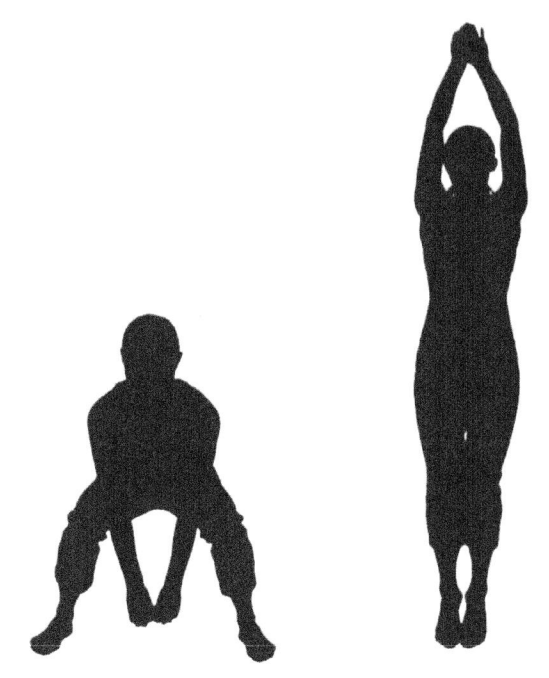

Dip knees in preparation to leap and then push upwards, as if you're pushing the floor away from you as you jump up. Swing arms upwards to help gain momentum.

Your upper body should stay as upright as possible. When you land, immediately squat down and jump up again. Repeat 5- 10 times.

Lean Legs Tip:

Getting the Most Out of Your Body-Weight Exercises

Body-weight exercises can be a good choice for beginners, when out on the road or when you're short of cash! Moves like push-ups, dips, squats, and lunges can help you work your body without the need of extra equipment.

However, remember the principle of overload: If you want your body to get stronger and fitter, you have to challenge it with more weight than it can handle. When the body-weight exercises get too easy, you'll need to add some type of resistance to increase the challenge [63].

For some more body-weight exercise ideas, visit:

http://exercise.about.com/library/bltravelworkout.htm

32. Standing Knee Hug

Targets: Thighs, calves ankles, hamstrings, hips, low back

Stand with feet together and arms by sides.

Move weight to one foot and put hand on that hip. Slowly pull knee of opposite leg up towards chest. Hug knee to chest with corresponding hand (as pictured).

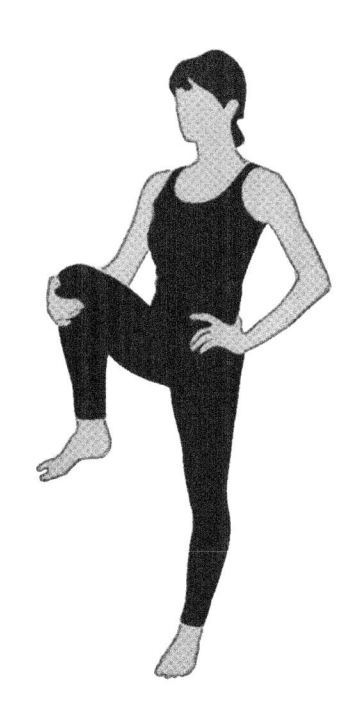

Stand tall, contracting muscles of standing leg and abs. Keep leg straight but don't lock knee. Keep hips straight forward and shoulders relaxed.

Hold for 30 seconds, lower foot and relax before repeating move on opposite side.

33. Side Knee Hug

Targets: Thighs, calves, ankles, hamstrings, core muscles

Stand with feet together and arms at sides. Shift weight to one foot. Bring corresponding hand to hip. Slowly draw knee of other leg up towards chest. Using corresponding hand, hug knee into chest.

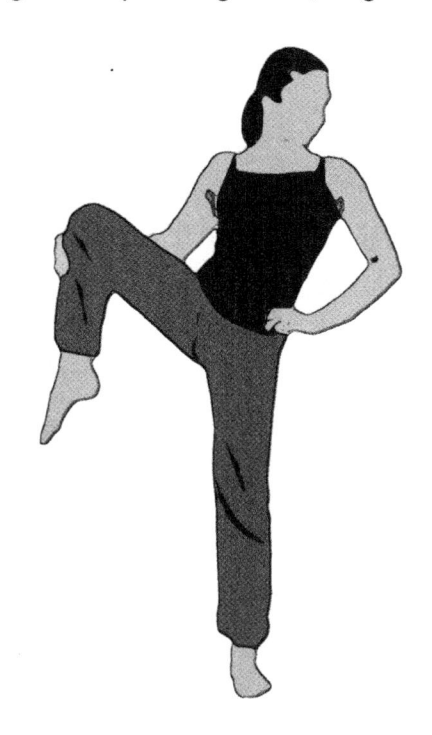

Pause for a few seconds, and if comfortable and steady, and can maintain a straight spine, use hand to help open knee to side (as pictured).

Let shin and foot hang just beneath knee. At the same time, engage muscles of other leg, but do not lock knee. Keep core tight to steady body and spine straight. Relax shoulders.

Maintain pose for 10 seconds, and then release pose, bringing knee back to middle, hugging it back into chest. Slowly lower foot to floor. Repeat pose on opposite side.

34. Front and Side Swings

Targets: Glutes, hips

Stand with arms crossed in front at shoulder height. With abs tight, raise one knee towards corresponding elbow.

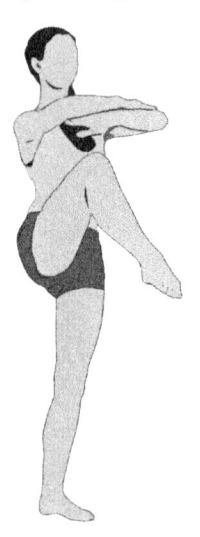

Next, swing both arms and knee out to side. Cross arms back in front, and knee back to corresponding elbow as before to complete rep.

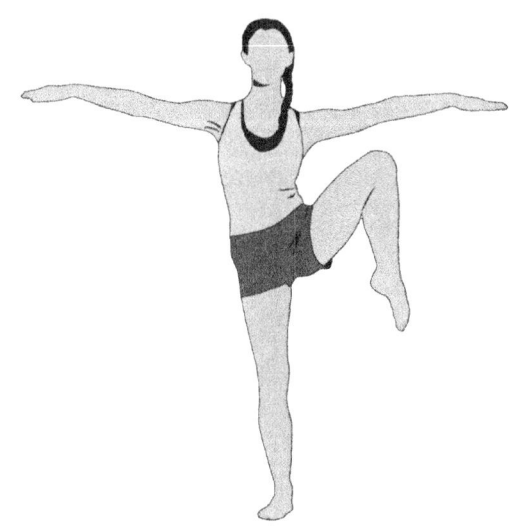

Repeat movement for 10 swings at a steady pace. Lower leg, and then repeat swings with opposite leg.

Lean Legs Tip:

How to Accelerate Fat Loss with Body-Weight Moves

One of the best ways to maximize fat loss with body-weight exercises is by using a technique call **metabolic resistance training (MRT)** [64].

MRT is similar to high intensity interval training (HIIT), in that it helps burn more calories post workout by raising levels of **EPOC** [65].

The goal of MRT is to help expend more energy — by burning calories and elevating metabolism — rather than building strength and muscle [66].

5 MRT Tricks to Help You Boost Post Workout Fat Burn

To maximize the 'after burn' effect of MRT, try these 5 techniques: [Bodyweight Strength Training Anatomy, Bret Contreras, pgs 168-169]

1. Use compound exercises, or exercises that work a lot of muscles at the same time [67].

2. **Alternate between lower and upper body exercises**: This allows your heart to continually transport blood throughout your body, and gives individual muscles a rest so they can recharge between stints [68].

3. Include whole-body exercises because they're excellent for raising the heart rate [69].

4. Use short rest periods between sets and exercises. Short rest periods, usually 30 seconds or less, release important fat-burning hormones, and allow you to burn more calories per minute [70] [71].

35. Prisoner Cycle Lunge

Targets: Core, thighs, glutes

Stand tall with feet together and fingers interlaced behind head (as pictured).

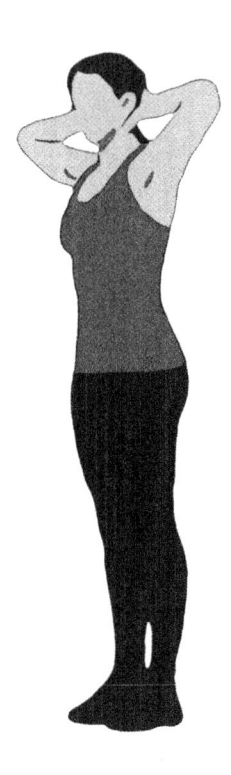

Step forward with one leg and drop into lunge.

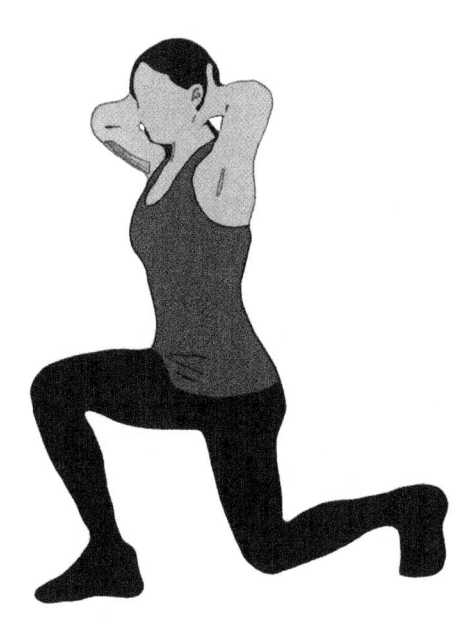

Reverse move, stepping into reverse lunge with leg to complete rep. Repeat move with opposite leg. Continue to move at a steady pace for 30-60 seconds, switching sides each time.

36. Ski Moguls

Targets: Glutes

Standing tall with feet together, squat down and swing arms back.

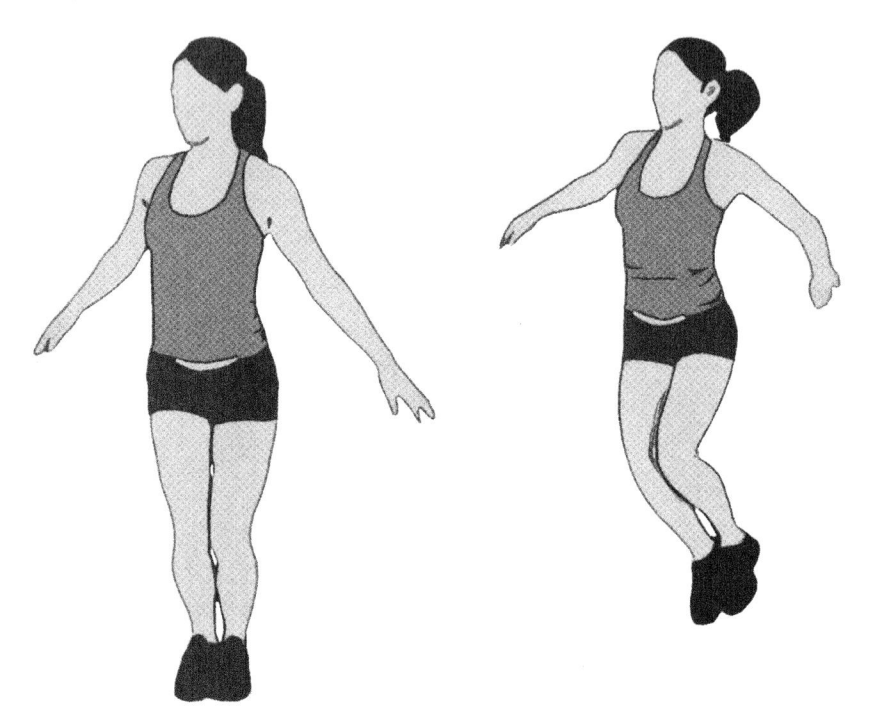

Jump across to one side while swinging arms forwards. Land softly with feet together. Repeat movement, squatting and jumping to other side.

Continue to move at a steady pace for 30-60 seconds, jumping from side to side each time.

37. Single Leg Heel Raises

Targets: Calves, quads, glutes

Start by standing on balls of foot and holding onto chair for balance. Place one foot behind heel of other foot.

Rise up on ball of one foot as high as is comfortable, and at the same time, bend knee of back leg (as pictured). Pause for a second, and then return to start. Repeat for 5 reps, and then switch sides.

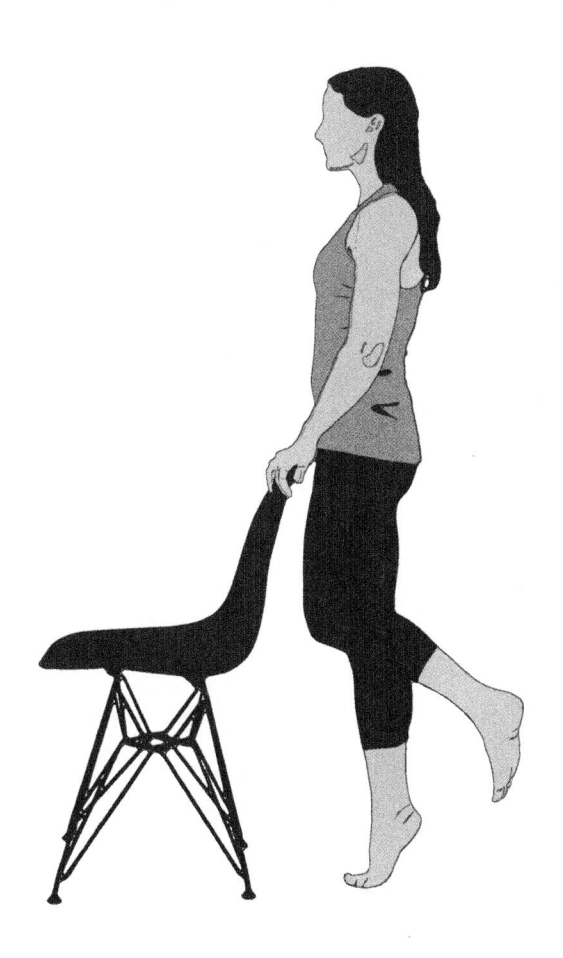

Section Seven: Floor Workouts

Lying floor exercises are a convenient and 'stress lite' way to work out your lower body. They're excellent for firming legs, plus floor exercises help target the powerful hard-to-reach muscles which engage abs, lift glutes and slim thighs — without placing tension on joints.

Pilates: The Ultimate 'Squat Free' Floor Workout for Sculpting Legs

If want to get those coveted shapelier pins without the squatting and lunging, then including some basic Pilates moves in your leg workouts is one way to go.

Though Pilates is primarily known as an exercise for building stronger core muscles, within its repertoire of over 500 moves are exercises for firming, shaping and strengthening legs. The Pilates method of working from the core when doing any movements also gives your spine, knees and hips a break, and helps your body work more efficiently. [72]

The Core Connection: How Using Your Abs Benefits Your Lower Body

Your abdominal muscles — plus the 29 muscles in and around your trunk and pelvis, and those of the hips, buttocks and lower back — are your core [73]. The creator of Pilates (Joe Pilates) referred to this as the *powerhouse*.

In Pilates, the deepest layers of your abdominal or powerhouse muscles are worked to completely realign and reshape your body. [74].

When all of the core muscles are at their most strongest, they provide support, stability, and added power to any strength training activity [75].

Pilates works many muscles together in one movement, instead of in isolation, to lengthen upwards and outwards. [76] [77]. Additionally, they are worked through a fuller range of motion.

This combination of stretching, strengthening and muscles working together prevents big muscles from getting too bulky, and helps you create a lean, toned body. [78], [79].

In this section you'll find a variety of lying floor exercises — side, prone (on abs) and supine (on back) — to help sculpt and shape the legs.

For a basic primer on Pilates, some good books for further reading are **Pilates For Dummies** By Ellie Herman and **Pilates: 50 Exercises to Strengthen, Lengthen, and Tone Your Muscles**, by Shirley Archer

38. Adductor Squeeze

Targets: Inner thighs

Start by lying flat on back, arms by sides, knees raised and bent, with a rolled towel or ball between them.

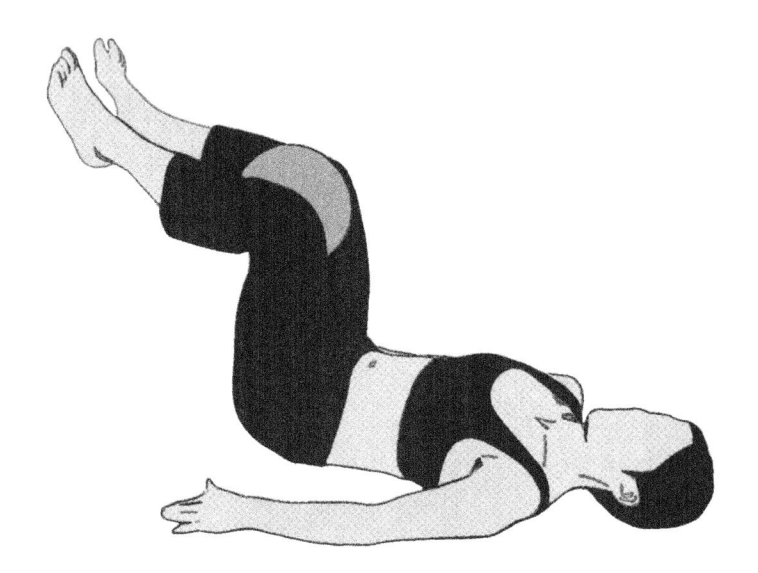

Slowly squeeze ball/towel between knees as hard as possible without pain, tightening inner thigh muscles. Hold for 5 seconds, and then relax muscles. Repeat exercise 10 times in total.

39. Crossed Legged Bridge

Targets: Glutes, core, back, chest

Start by lying on back, arms at sides, knees bent and feet flat on floor. Cross one leg over other, resting foot on knee.

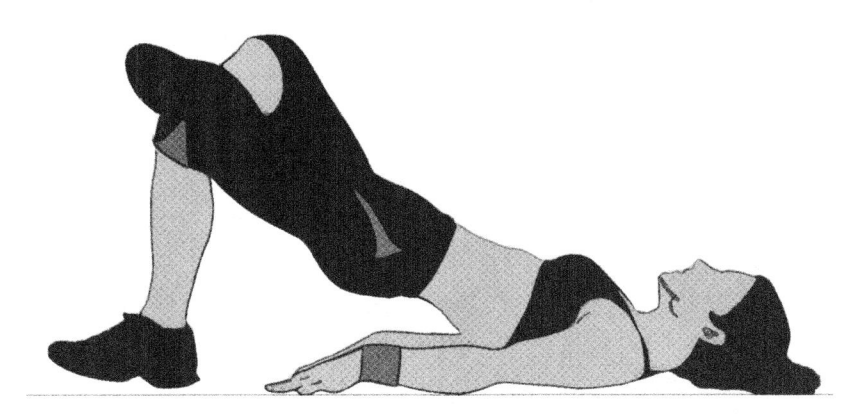

Lift hips upwards, pause for second, contracting glutes and hamstrings at top of move, and then lower. Do not overarch spine.

Repeat move for one set of 10 reps. Repeat for another 10 reps if desired.

40. Single Leg Circles

Targets: Thighs, glutes, core

Lying on back and arms at sides, have one foot flat on floor, the other leg extended towards ceiling with toes pointed.

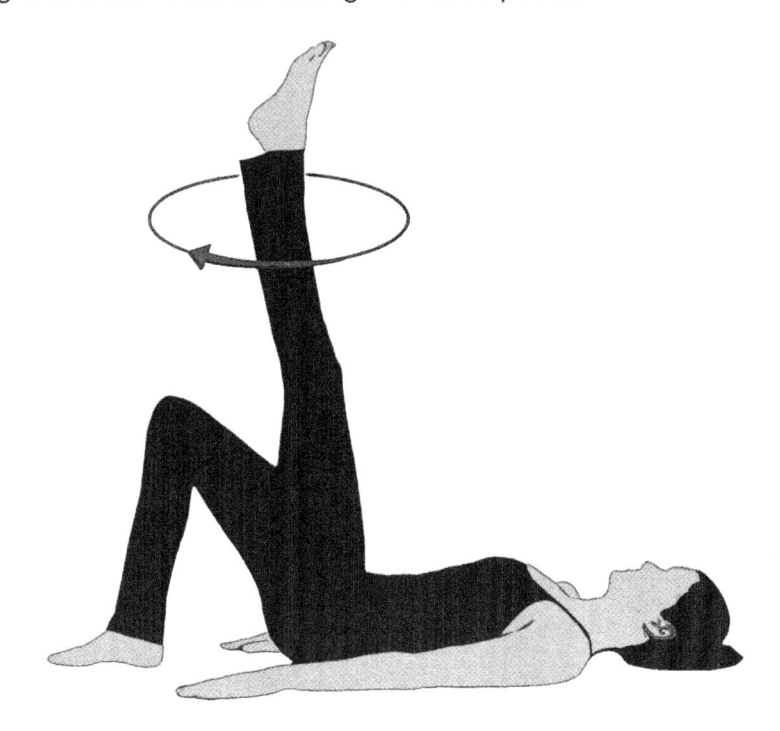

Pausing for 10 seconds, rotate leg from hip in small circles, keeping abs tight throughout. Steadily inhale and exhale as you perform exercise.

Do 5 circles in one direction and then another 5 the opposite way. Switch legs and repeat.

Harder: Perform as once before, but this time, straighten other leg out on floor, while extending other leg towards ceiling.

41. Single Leg Kick

Targets: Hamstrings, core, back

Lie on belly, legs extended behind at hip width distance, and slightly lifted off floor. Prop upper body onto forearms at shoulder width distance.

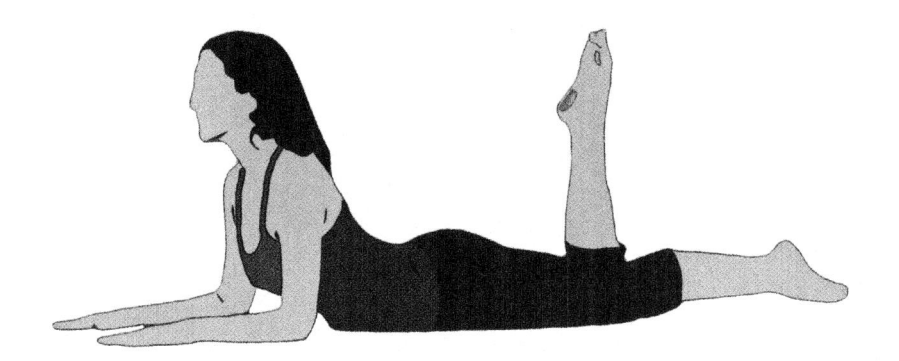

With abs muscles tight, kick one leg towards back and return it to lifted position. Repeat move with other leg. Continue to alternate between legs at a steady pace for a 10 second rep. Relax and then repeat exercise for another 10 seconds.

42. Swimming

Targets: Back, shoulders, glutes

Lie on belly with arms reaching overhead and legs straight. Extend one leg and opposite arm out and up towards ceiling (as pictured).

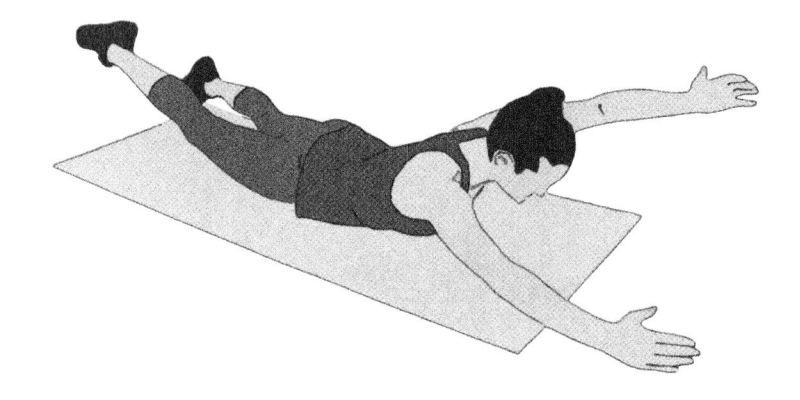

Change arm and leg quickly without losing balance of upper body.

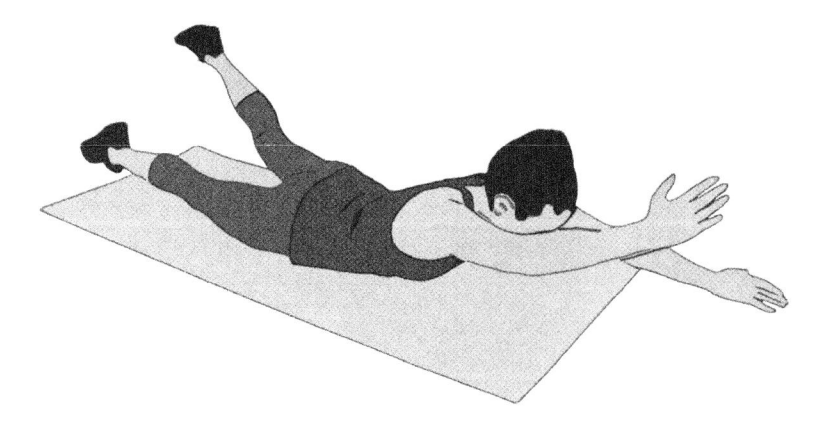

Continue to move as quickly as possible without losing balance between two sides of body. Maintain 'swimming' motion for 10-15 seconds before relaxing. Repeat once more, if desired.

43. Bird-Dog

Targets: Abs, back, glutes and hips

Get down on hands and knees. Making sure are abs fully engaged, extend one arm and opposing leg, so they're in line with torso. Hold pose for 7-8 seconds and then return to starting position.

Make sure that back remains still throughout when performing this exercise. Do 2–3 sets of 8–15 reps.

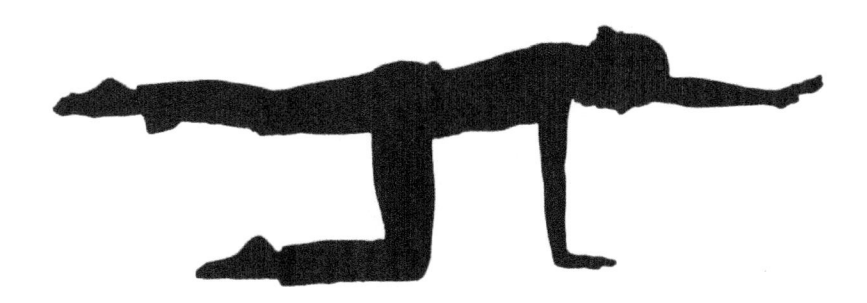

44. Single Leg Stretch

Targets: Core, lower back, hip flexors, pelvis

Start by resting on back, knees bent, arms by sides with palms down.

As you lift head and shoulders off mat, draw one leg towards chest with hands, while extending other leg out (at 45 degrees).

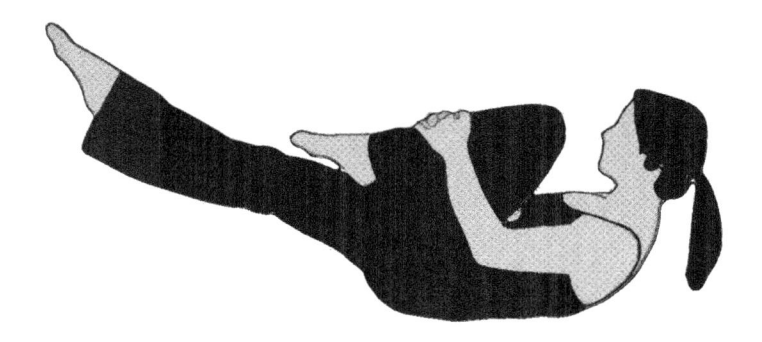

Hold for 5 seconds, and then switch legs and repeat move. Continue to alternate between legs for a total of 10 reps.

45. Hip Raise/Glute Bridge

Targets: Lower back, glutes, core, hamstrings, hips

Lie on back with feet placed on foam roller. With core tight, drive hips upwards, then lift one leg until parallel with thigh.

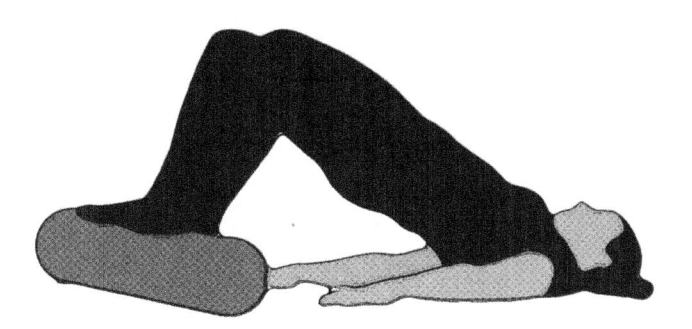

Hold pose 10 seconds, and then slowly lower body and leg. Do a total of five 10 second reps, then change legs and repeat.

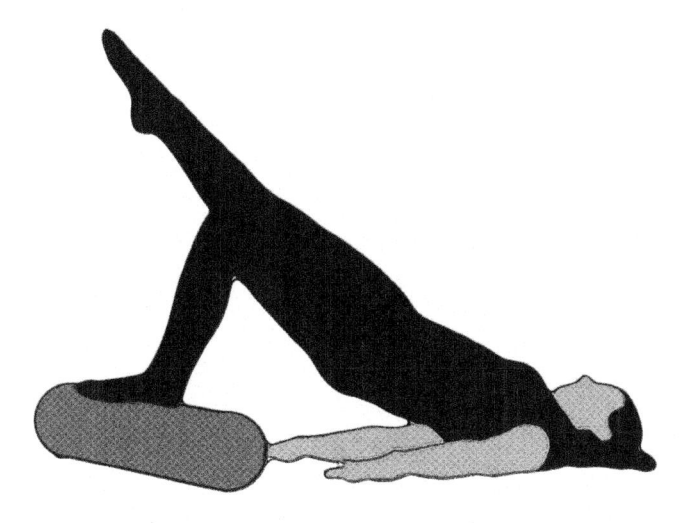

Section Eight: Knee Strengthening Workouts

We ask a lot of our knees. Whether it's kicking, jumping or a pummeling during a jog, our knees willing oblige by winding, bending and absorbing the impact. But amazingly, the structure for the knee is incredibly fragile.

Knee Anatomy 101

Compared to other joints in the body, such as the ankle or hip, the one in the knee connecting the thigh bone (femur) and shin bone (tibia) is essentially a shallow and unstable hinge. In a manner of speaking, an imperfect fit [80] [81].

Whereas the hip joint has a ball-in-socket design and the ankle joint neatly slides in, support for the knee depends on small ligaments (joining bone to bone) and tendons (joining muscle to bone) to hold it together [82].

Furthermore, the hamstring muscles are responsible for the knee's bending action, while the quad muscles straighten it [83].

Why Stronger Thighs Equals Stronger Knees

The quads, found in the front of your thighs, are one of the most important muscle groups because you engage them whenever you walk, run and jump.

They're also the most powerful muscles for keeping your knee moving properly, [83] and control how much pressure they (and kneecaps) feel with every step [84].

Any imbalances or damage sustained in the quads greatly affects the knee. Therefore, building stronger quad muscles is an essential key to providing stability to the knee joints' delicate set-up, and protects them from injury.

In fact, research has shown that stronger quads can help cartilage loss in the knees — a symptom of osteoarthritis [85].

Note that even if you're runner or a frequent walker, you *still* need to supplement these activities with a good strength building program. Put side by side, activities such as Pilates, yoga, weight lifting and biking, will do a much better job at developing quad muscle power.

Why Better Flexibility Also Means Stronger Knees

In **105 Stretching Exercises for Women**, we touch upon why quad stretches are one of the 10 most important stretches you should do.

For your quad muscles, keeping them flexible is as important as strengthening them, to prevent them from becoming short and tight. Even if you don't strengthen quads, they will become short if not worked through their full ROM [86].

With little or no stretching, the soft tissues of body parts simply conform to the shapes in which they spend the most time [87]. And if you seldom stretch the quads, you will lose the ability to fully flex or bend the knee.

For some simple and useful post exercise stretches, please refer back to **section two**. Alternatively, **105 Stretching Exercises for Women** has a wide selection of stretches for the major lower body muscles.

Some simple post exercise stretching tips:

- When performing stretches, a general guideline is to hold each pose for 30 seconds and then switch sides.

- Keep your breathing soft and controlled throughout all of the exercises.

- Take note at what point you feel the stretch or where you stop when performing each exercise. This will give you a general indication of your current level of ROM.

- Perform the stretches at least twice a day, 5-6 times a week for the greatest improvement.

- Do not force or overdo a stretch beyond the point of comfort.

In this section is selection of low impact thigh focused strengtheners to help build healthier and stronger knees.

46. Tree Pose

Targets: Quads, core, hips, abs

Standing up straight, bend one knee and place sole of foot on inner thigh or calf. Clasp hands together in prayer in middle of chest.

Reach arms up overhead, hold pose for 10-20 seconds and then release. Repeat pose with opposite leg.

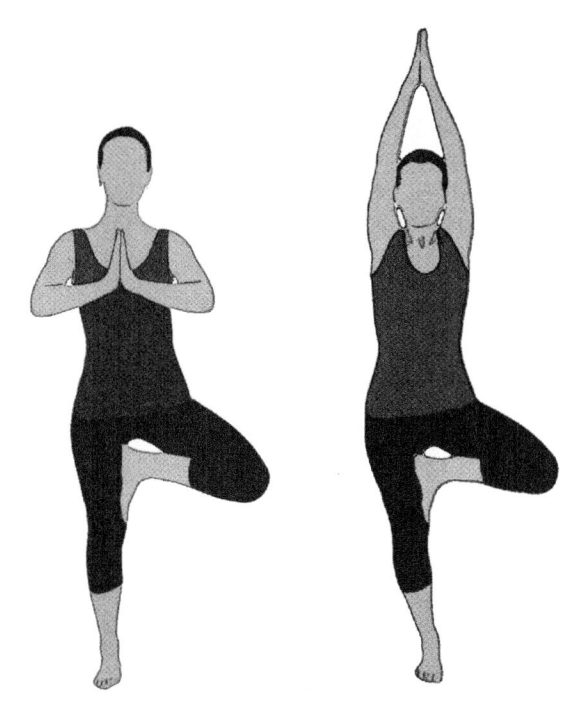

Easier: Perform move as described before, however put foot on inside of ankle, with toes lightly touching floor.

47. Bridge with Straight Leg Raise

Targets: Hips, quads, glutes, abs

Start by lying on back, arms at sides, knees bent and feet flat on floor. Lift hips upwards, until body is parallel from knee to shoulders.

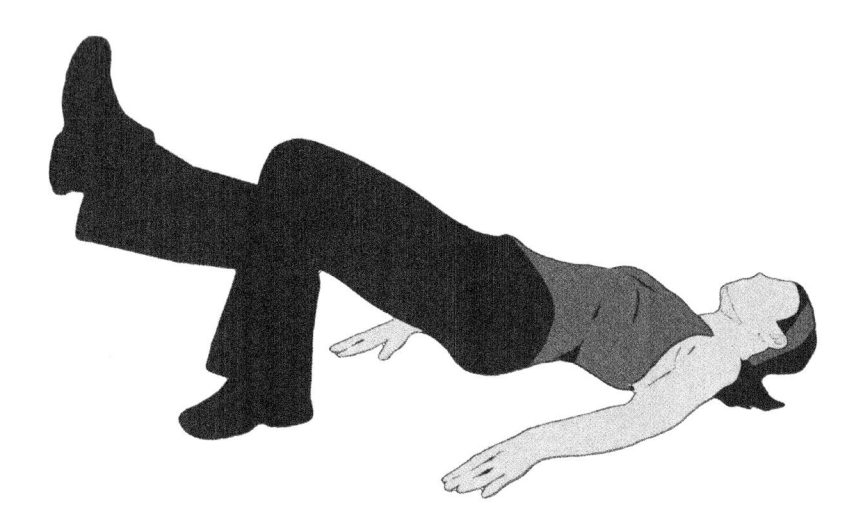

As you rise, extend one leg in line with body. Pause for second, contracting glutes and hamstrings at top of move, and then lower. Do not overarch spine.

Repeat move for one set of 10 reps. Repeat for another 10 reps if desired.

48. Warrior II

Targets: Quads, hamstrings, glutes, hips, back, chest, and shoulders

Start with feet together and arms at sides. Take large step out to one side. Rotate one heel slightly outwards and turn other leg, so as foot points outwards and hips face forwards.

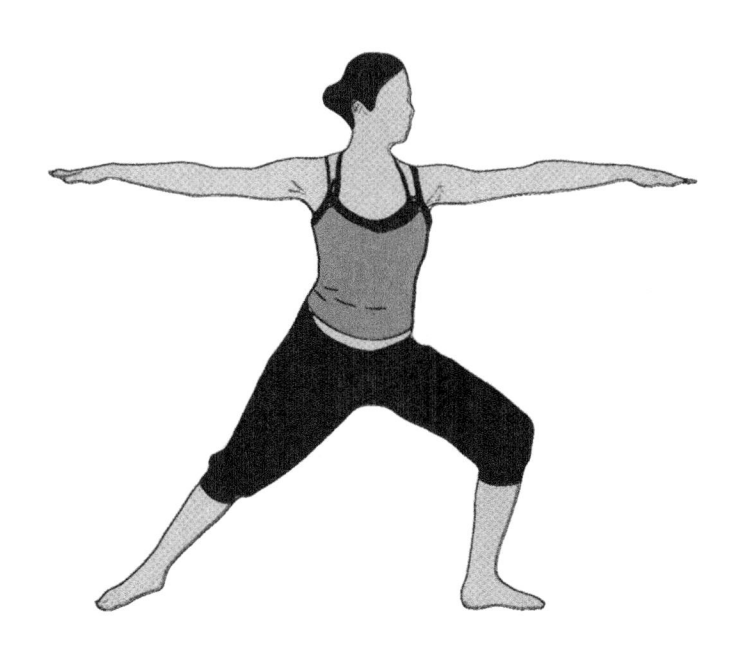

Bring arms up to shoulder height and stretch out to sides.

Bend knee until it's at a right angle, and then look out along one extended arm towards fingertips (as pictured). Hold for 5 seconds, and then step back to starting position before repeating pose on other side.

49. Modified Side Angle Pose

Targets: legs, knees, ankles, arms, abs

With feet wide apart, turn left foot out 90 degrees and other at 45 degrees. Bend right knee, making sure that kneecap is just over ankle.

Place right elbow on bended right knee — or put palm of hand on shin (as pictured). Extend left arm alongside head, forming a slanting pose from foot to arm.

Hold pose for 30 seconds. Return to starting position and then repeat on other side.

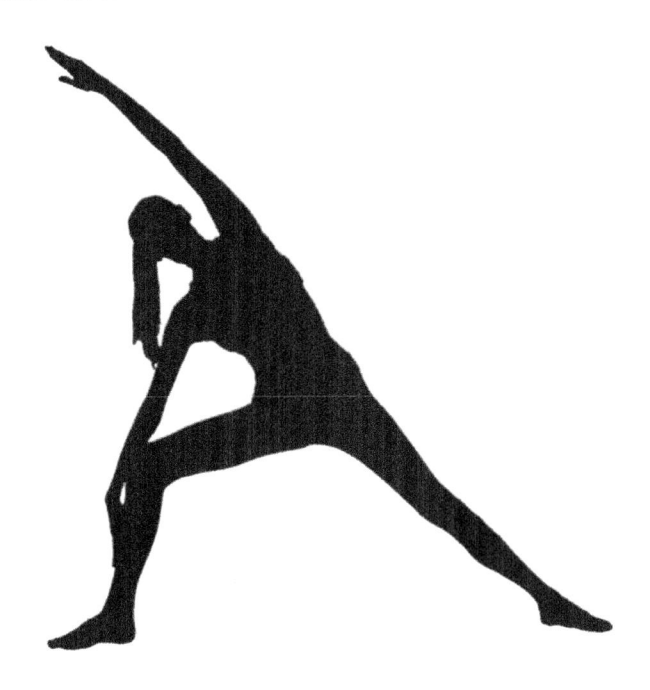

50. Standing Knee Bends (Shallow Squats)

Targets Glutes, quads, hamstrings

Stand with feet at shoulder width distance.

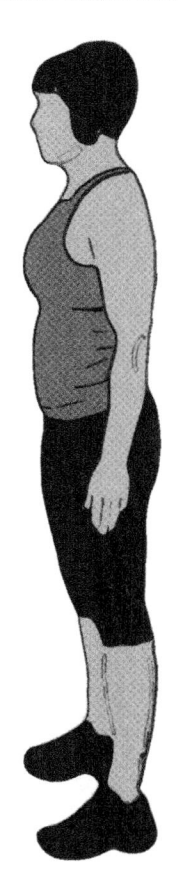

Slowly bend knees into shallow squat, making sure heels remain on floor and knees do not extend over toes. Pause for second, and then slowly rise to standing.

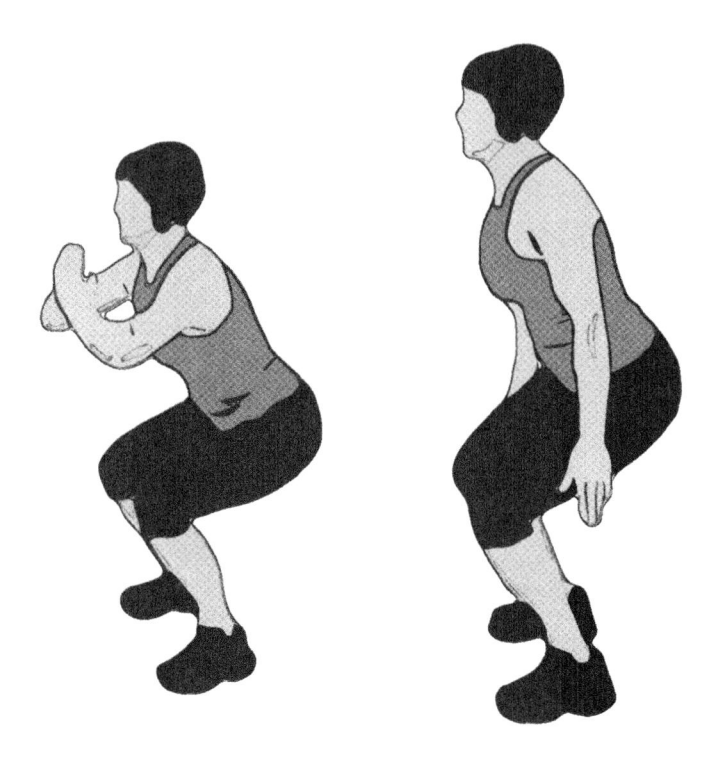

As you perform squat, keep back straight and tighten glute muscles. Do 10 reps.

51. The Plank

Targets: Core, glutes, arms (also back and quadriceps)

Support body on all fours by planting palms flat down, knees lifted, balancing firmly on toes and hands directly beneath shoulders.

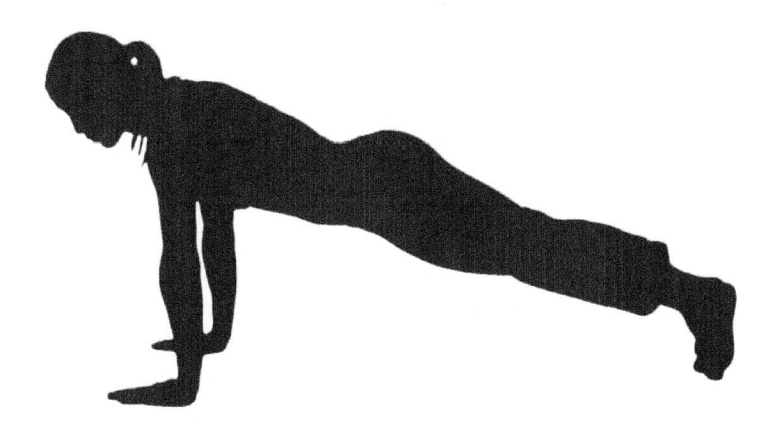

As you hold pose, keep abs tight and body aligned from head to heels. Hold position for 30 seconds (minimum 15 seconds!). Release pose and lower body. Repeat once more.

Lean Legs Tip:

6 Ways to Keep Your Knees Healthy

In addition to strengthening the surrounding muscles, there are a number of simple measures you can take to keep your knees healthy:

1. Take Glucosamine Plus Chondroitin:

Glucosamine is a nutritional supplement that can help reduce mild pain from arthritis and other musculoskeletal pain. Chondroitin, also a nutritional supplement, is a component of normal cartilage and is often used in combination with glucosamine.

When taken together with chondroitin, glucosamine is thought to help knee pain caused by wear and tear or even osteoarthritis, by keeping cartilage supple and in good supply [88] [89].

2. Take Calcium and Vitamin D:

According to medical experts, everyone (especially women over fifteen years old) should make sure they're getting **1500 mg of calcium**, and **400 I.U. of vitamin D** a day [90]. Both calcium and Vitamin D are both essential to building healthy bones.

Vitamin D regulates many normal body functions and tissues, maintains cardiovascular health, and helps your body use calcium more efficiently.

3. Maintain A Healthy Weight:

Osteoarthritis is caused by wear and tear. Extra weight puts far more pressure on your joints just through everyday activities. In fact, your knees absorb **6 to 7 times** your body weight just by going down the stairs! [91]

4. Use The Right Equipment When Exercising:

For example, get fitted for your bike or buy proper shoes. Minor things, such as wearing worn-out walking sneakers or ill fitting footwear, begin to add up and cause pain as we age [92].

5. Drink Plenty Of Water:

Keeping properly hydrated is one of the key essentials in preventing injury. Water is a vital part of good muscle contraction, and if muscles aren't contracting efficiently, you'll feel weaker, experience cramping and put yourself at greater risk of injury [93].

6. Build Your Training Slowly:

Most excessive injuries are from doing too much, too fast, and/or too often. Improper training or performing intense activities without carefully easing into them first will get you hurt. Even if you're in good shape, be careful not to have unrealistic expectations for your body, and don't do more than your body can handle [94].

52. Prone Plank

Targets: Core, glutes, arms (also back and quadriceps)

In a horizontal position, support body on toes and forearms. Your shoulders should be a little over elbows and feet a few inches apart.

With back, glutes and head parallel hold this position for 30 seconds and then release.

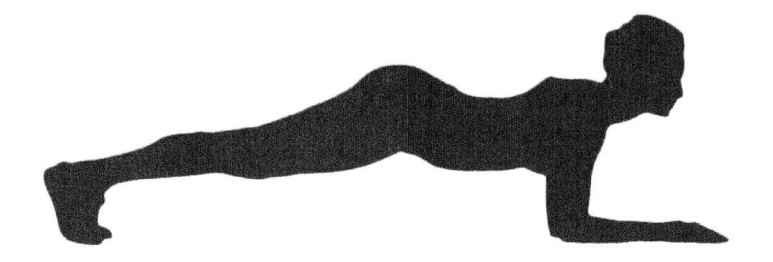

53. Standing Cradle Leg Stretch

Targets: Glutes, hamstrings, hips, quads

Begin in a hip width stance and arms by sides. Raise one leg, bend knee and draw foot towards opposite hip, rotating inner ankle towards ceiling.

Next, hold ankle with one hand and hold bottom part of foot with other hand (as pictured).

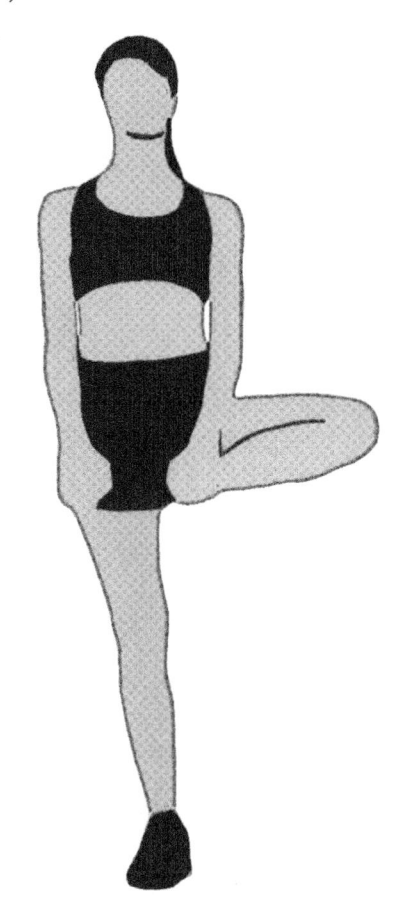

Gently draw whole leg upwards until you feel a gentle stretch. Hold for 10 seconds and then release and lower leg. Repeat stretch with other leg.

Section Nine: Pregnancy Leg Workouts

Toning legs and glutes during pregnancy is an ideal time, as it can help you identify different muscle groups and potential problem areas [95].

Strong legs and glutes are also going to be a big plus during the birthing process. They'll help position you comfortably for labour and for birth, and by increasing both strength and tone during pregnancy, you'll aid in making labour *a lot* easier [96].

As noted back in **section four**, any added fuel needed to feed the baby will come in the form of fat cells, which accumulate mostly around the upper thighs (including the gluteal area) during pregnancy [97] [98].

Breastfeeding and exercise are going to be some of the best ways to burning this extra fat.

General Guidelines for Exercising During Pregnancy

Research shows that pregnant women can safely continue to exercise at whatever fitness level they are presently at. Though the stipulation is not to overdo it. The duration of your exercise sessions does depend on what you did before your pregnancy, according to exercise experts [99].

While it's not been conclusively established as to whether it's safe for expectant mothers to exercise for an hour or more, the general consensus is to keep your workout to **45 minutes or less** (35 minutes if you're a beginner). This includes warm-up and cool-down periods [100].

Some further recommendations also include that you:

- Exercise at least 3 times a week.

- Do modest activity such as like walking or swimming on most, if not all, days of the week.

- Limit intense activities (e.g. running or aerobics) to 4 times per week.

Lower Body Strength Training During Pregnancy

Though some form of cardio fitness is a must as part of your workouts, strength training is especially needed when you're pregnant to complete your fitness routine. This is because building bigger and stronger muscles will:

- Help your body to increase its metabolism, as muscles burn more calories than fat.

- Fuel your body during hard and long physical challenges — like childbirth.

- **Store more reserves of glycogen.** This comes in handy if you have to stay in the same positions for long amounts of time come labour day!

Home Gym Equipment Basics for the Expectant Mother

Some basic recommendations for equipment include some hand-held free weights, an exercise band, a mat or cushion for protection and some sturdy furniture for support. To experience the benefits from strength training, you should try to do some twice a week. Any more than this is not advised.

A final note is that with the exception of squats and the pelvic rock, you should stop strength training 2 weeks before your baby's due date. Exercising after this point isn't suggested, as the strain on your body will be counter-productive.

Some of the advice provided in this chapter was based on information from the book '**Nine Months Strong: Shaping Up for Labor and Delivery and the Toughest Physical Day of Your Life**', **by** Karen Bridson and Karin Blakemore.

NB: Though this chapter contains a compilation of exercises considered to be safe to perform during and after pregnancy, **please consult a health professional** before starting any kind of strength training program.

54. Downward Facing Dog

Targets: arms, shoulders, chest, legs, abs

Get down on all fours, with wrists a few inches in front of shoulders.

Part knees at hip width distant and curl toes under. Pushing equally into palms, lift knees off the floor. Raise sitting bone upwards so that you form a reversed "V" (as pictured).

Slowly straighten knees and lift heels off floor without locking them in position. Gradually inch torso towards thighs, until arms are aligned with ears. Relax head, but don't let it dangle.

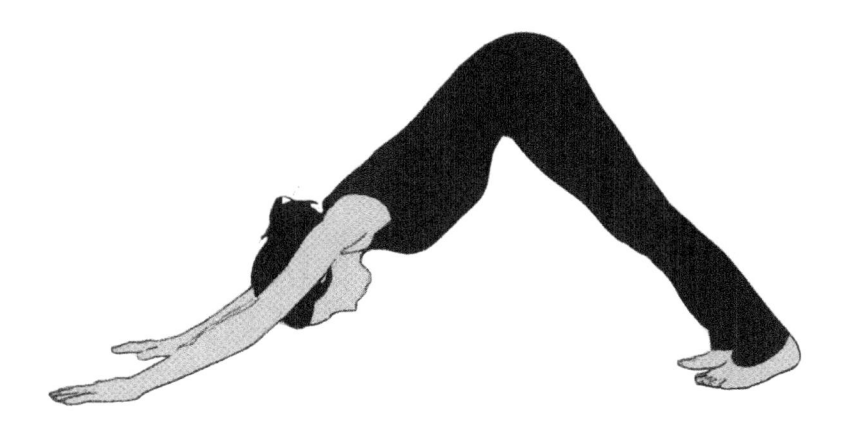

Hold pose for as long as you can, keeping hips lifted and pushing firmly into hands. Bend knees to floor and then rest.

The same move can be performed using a chair as support for arms.

55. Side Leg Lifts with Shoulder Press

Targets: Glutes, hips, thighs, shoulders

Stand with feet at hip width distance, resistance-band looped around ankles, dumbbell in each hand, arms at shoulder height and elbows bent.

Slowly lift one leg out to side as you lift arms above head. Return to start and repeat with opposite leg to compete 1 rep. Do 10 reps, alternating between legs.

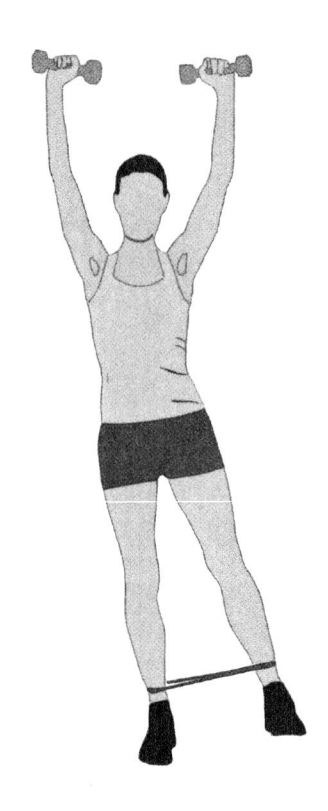

56. Squats to Side Leg Lifts with One Arm Lateral/Front Raises

Targets: Shoulders, delts, back, outer thighs, glutes, quads

Standing beside chair with feet close together, hold dumbbell in one hand and rest other hand on chair for support.

First phase:

As you lower into shallow squat, slowly lift dumbbell to shoulder height. Hold for second at top of lift, and then slowly lower dumbbell and return to standing.

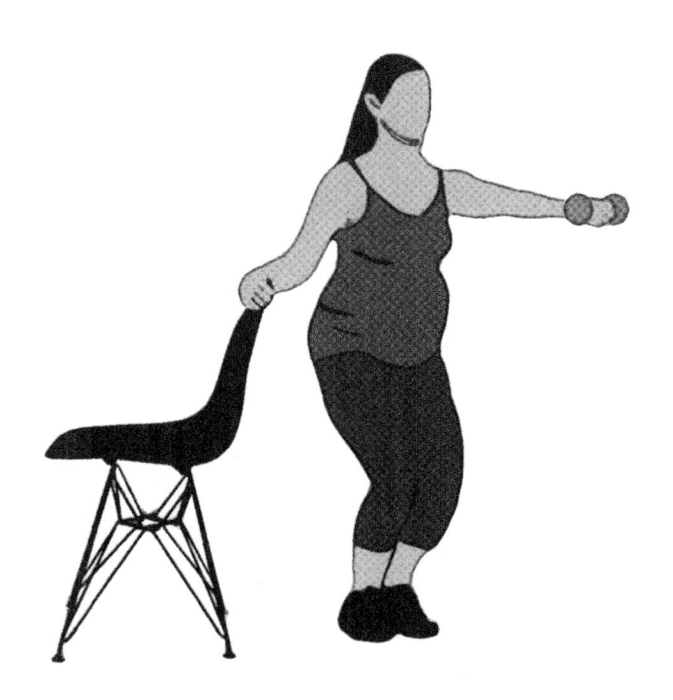

Second phase:

As you return to standing, slowly lift one leg and dumbbell out to side to shoulder level. Hold for second at top of lift, and then slowly lower leg and arm to complete 1 rep.

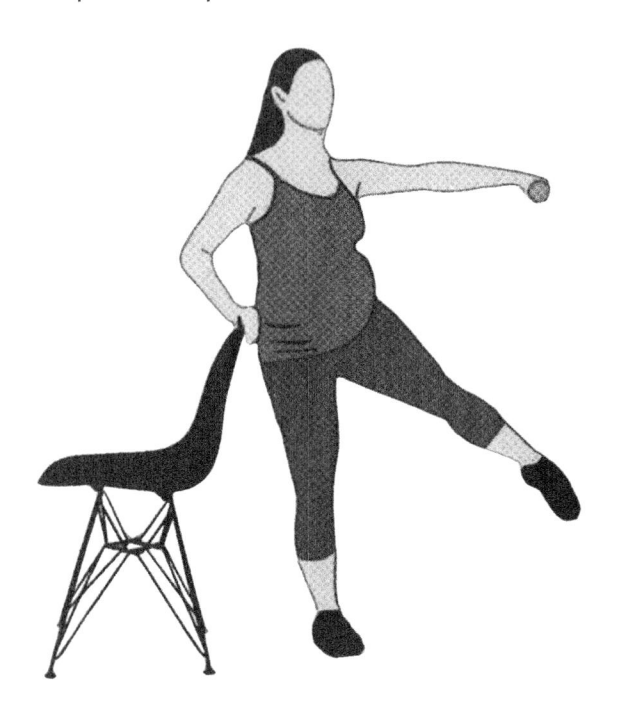

Continue exercise at a steady pace for 10 reps, alternating between first and second phase on each rep.

Lean Legs Tip:

How to Stop Night Leg Cramps

Many pregnant women suffer from leg cramps, particularly at night. Well-toned and strengthened muscles will be less prone to this problem, but a good stretch of the lower leg just before bed will help lessen the likelihood of night cramps. Additionally, plenty of calcium and potassium as part of your diet, and as already mentioned, drinking lots of water can also help prevent cramps [101].

57. Floor Leg Lifts

Targets: Hip and thighs

Lie on one side with arm resting on floor, elbow bent, and place other hand on hip. Extend legs with knees slightly bent (or straight) and stack one on top of other.

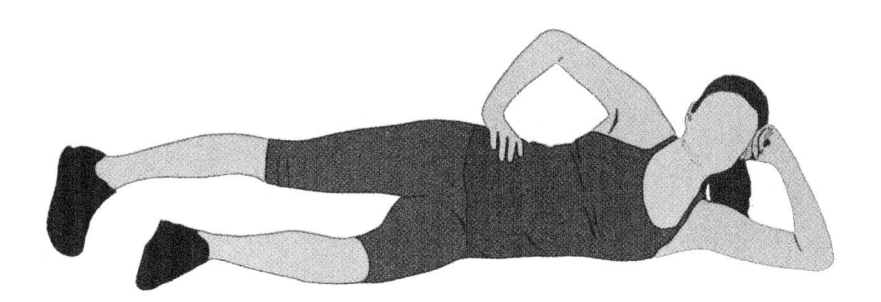

Lift top leg as high as possible, and then lower and float leg just above floor in front of bottom leg.

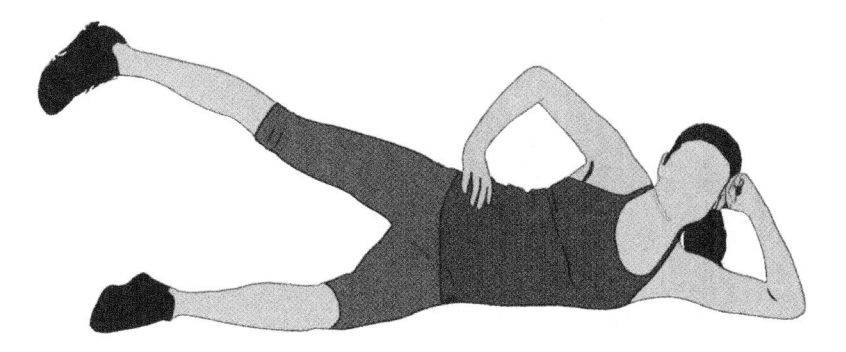

Continue to lift and lower top leg, without foot touching floor between reps. Perform 10 reps and switch sides and repeat once more to complete exercise.

58. Resistance Band Side Twists

Targets: Glutes, hips, thighs, waist

Tie one end of exercise band to piece of sturdy furniture, holding other end of band with both hands along with a dumbbell.

As you step one foot crosswise behind other foot, bend both knees, and then swing band and dumbbell down across body (as pictured).

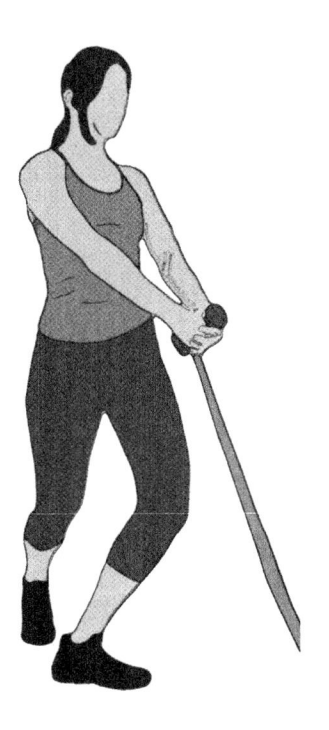

As you return to standing, bring back leg parallel to other leg, and then turn upper body to one side (as pictured) to complete rep. Do for 10 reps and then repeat on opposite side.

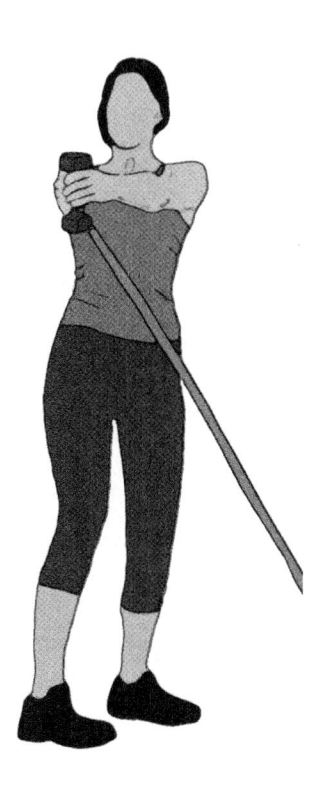

59. Standing Glutes Back Kicks

Targets: Glutes, hamstrings

Stand with exercise band strapped around ankles and with hands on hips. Kick one foot behind you to stretch band, tightening glute muscles at top of kick. Return to start and then repeat back kick. Do for 10 reps, and then back kick with other leg for 10 more reps.

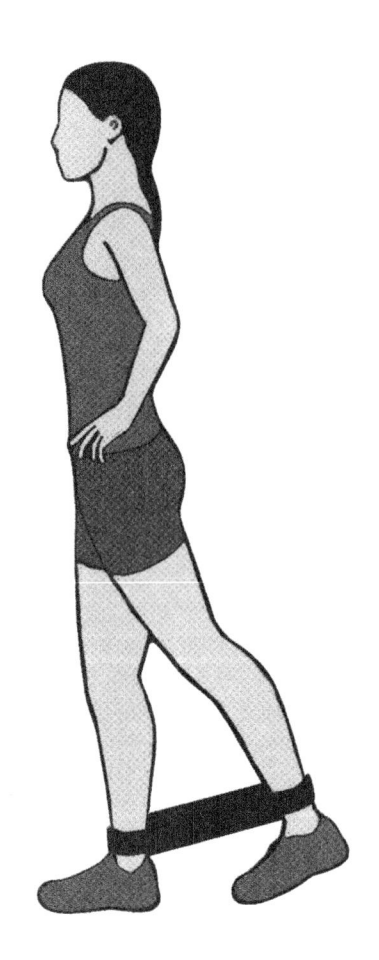

60. Lateral Walks

Targets: Hips

Start by lowering into shallow squat, feet at hip width distance, with exercise band strapped around thighs, just above knees.

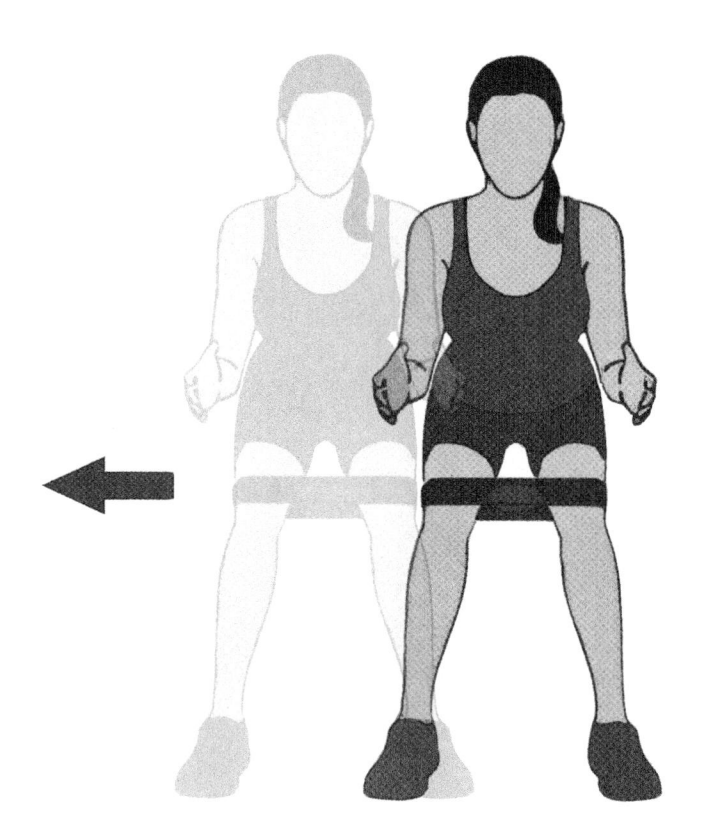

With one foot, step to one side slightly wider than shoulder width distance. Hold pose for few seconds. Step other foot to return to width of starting position (hips width).

Take 3 more steps in same direction, repeating sequence of movements as described, pausing for a few seconds between each step.

Return to width of starting position, and then repeat same sequence of movements in opposite direction to complete 1 rep. Do 5-10 reps.

61. Goblet Squat

Targets: Quads, calves, glutes, hamstrings

Start by standing wider than shoulder width distance, holding dumbbell down between legs.

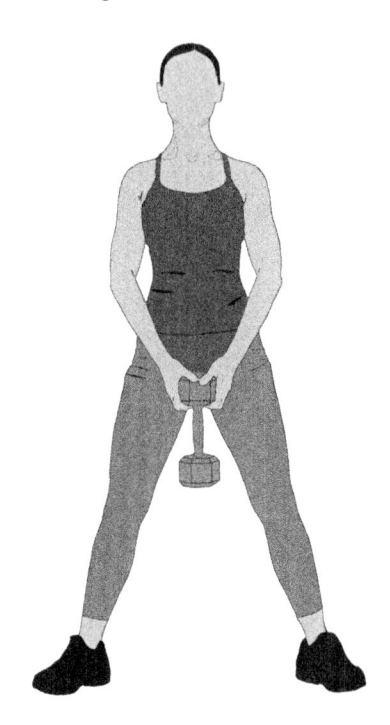

Squat down, lowering dumbbell between legs, keeping chest and head up, and back straight throughout.

At bottom position, hold for few seconds, and then return to start. Perform 10 reps to complete 1 set. Repeat another set, if desired.

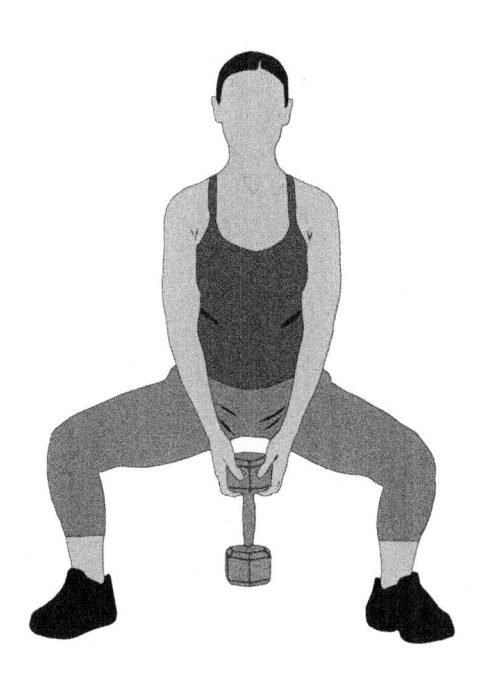

Index of Exercises

A

Adductor Squeeze, 89
Ankle Flex, 13

B

Back Stretch on Fitness Ball, 23
Bird-Dog, 94
Bridge, 67
Bridge with Straight Leg Raise, 101

C

Calf Raises, 44
Crossed Legged Bridge, 90

D

Dead Lifts, 59
Downward Facing Dog, 114

F

Floor Leg Lifts, 118
Forward Lunges, 48
Frog Hops, 41
Front and Side Swings, 81

G

Goblet Squat, 123

H

High Knees, 28
Hip Lifts, 40
Hip Raise, 96
Hip Swings, 26

I

Inner Thigh Lifts, 37
Inner Thigh Stretch, 17

J

Jump Squats, 77

K

Kickbacks, 55
Kickbacks with Resistance Band, 56
Knee thrust to Front Kick, 52

L

Lateral Walks, 122
Leg Presses, 73
Lying Hamstring Curl, 62
Lying Leg Extensions, 24
Lying Piriformis Stretch, 18

M

Marching on the Spot, 29
Modified Side Angle Pose, 103

O

One Leg Balance, 33
One Legged Squats, 57
Outer Thigh Lifts, 38

P

Plies, 43
Power Skips, 25
Prisoner Cycle Lunge, 83
Prone Plank, 109

Q

Quad Stretch, 16

R

Resistance Band Side Twists, 119

S

Shin and Ankle Stretches, 20
Shoulder Width Squats, 58
Side Kick Squats, 50
Side Kicks, 54
Side Knee Hug, 80
Side Leg Lifts with Shoulder Press, 115
Side Step-outs with Knee Raise, 35
Single Leg Circles, 91
Single Leg Heel Raises, 86
Single Leg Kick, 92
Single Leg Stretch, 95
Single Leg Wall Squats, 72
Sitting Knee Lifts, 63
Sitting Walks, 69
Ski Moguls, 85
Spilt Squats, 70
Squats to Side Leg Lifts, 116
Standing Calf Stretches, 15
Standing Cradle Leg Stretch, 110
Standing Full Body Stretch, 21
Standing Glutes Back Kicks, 121
Standing Hamstring Stretch, 19
Standing Knee Bends, 104
Standing Knee Hug, 79
Standing Knee Lifts, 64
Standing Leg Swings/Kicks, 68
Step-ups with Arm Raises, 36
Straight Leg Kicks, 27
Supported Lean Back, 74
Swimming, 93

T

Table Top Balance on Fitness Ball, 34

The Plank, 106
Toe Balances, 14
Tree Pose, 100

W

Wall Squats, 71
Warrior, 102

Special Bonus

Free Chapter of 105 Stretching Exercises for Women: One Minute Moves to Help You Get Limber, Stronger, Faster

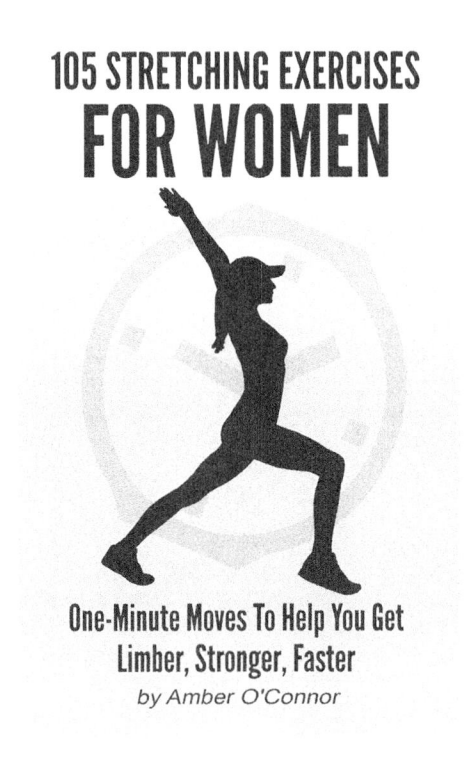

105 STRETCHING EXERCISES FOR WOMEN

One-Minute Moves To Help You Get Limber, Stronger, Faster

by Amber O'Connor

Want to know:

- The best lower back stretches that can help relieve pain - as suggested by top medical experts?

- The stealth bad habit almost all are guilty of, why it's the biggest cause of most body pain woes, and the upper/lower body flexibility moves that can help relieve them?

- Which moves can help you quickly regain flexibility, limber up tense muscles and deeply target hamstrings, the back, calves and other key areas?

- How foam roller stretches can help relieve tension and soothe sore muscles, plus how to target your whole body with the right moves.

- **Plus.....**some of the best gentle morning, noon and bedtime stretching moves to help wake you up, perk you up and chill you out?

If you answered yes to all of these questions, then get instant access now to **105 Stretching Exercises for Women: One Minute Moves to Help You Get Limber, Stronger, Faster.**

With a wide selection of clearly illustrated moves that can be done almost anywhere and at anytime of the day, this easy to follow guide is perfect for women who want to expand their flexibility beyond what they can currently do — and stay agile.

Download a free chapter of this book now at:

http://www.oneminutemovesbooks.com/freechapters.html

References

1-2. Bone Building Body Shaping Workout: Strength Health Beauty In Just 16, by Joyce L. Vedral, pg 87

3-5. 42-44 Strength Programs for Older Adults - Exercise ETC

6. Bounce Your Body Beautiful, Liz Applegate, Ph.D

7, 10, 12. Lewis-McCormick, Irene. A Woman's Guide to Muscle and Strength. Human Kinetics 1, 2012, pgs 4-5

8. Pagano, Joan. Strength Training Exercises for Women. Dorling Kindersley Ltd, 2014, pg 87

9, 11 Pedal Away Your Spare Tire by Selene Yeager, Bicycling May 2006, pg 118

13. 28-day Body Shapeover, by Brad Schoenfeld, pg 3

14-15 Bornstein, Adam. The Women's Health Big Book of Abs: Sculpt a Lean, Sexy Stomach in Just 4 Weeks! Rodale, 2012, pg 22

16-19. Women's Health Sep 2008, Stretching the Truth by Lisa Ann Smith, pg 146

20. Self Myofascial Release, http://www.sport-fitness-advisor.com

21. Get Moving! Live Better, Live Longer, Ruth K. Anderson, pg 28

22. The Metabolism Miracle: 3 Easy Steps to Regain Control of Your Weight, By Diane Kress, pg 156

23-28. Weight Training For Dummies, Georgia Rickard, Liz Neporent, Suzanne Schlosberg

29. 8 Minutes in the Morning to Lean Hips and Thin Thighs, Jorge Cruise, pg 14

30, 32-33, 38. Healing with Food By Anjali Mukherjee M. D. (A. M)

31, 34-37, 97. Hot Hips and Fabulous Thighs: Look Great in Just 6 Weeks, Ellington Darden, pg 18, 20

39. Ebony Aug 2000, Kimberly Davis, pg 36

40 -42 Bring It!: The Revolutionary Fitness Plan for All Levels That Burns Fat, Tony Horton, p161

43. Women's Health Sep 2007, Mike Mejia, pg 106

44-45. The Prevention Get Thin Get Young Plan, Selene Yeager, Bridget Doherty, pg 344

46-48. The Fat Burn Revolution: Boost Your Metabolism and Burn Fat Fast By Julia Buckley

49-50, 52. Sculpt Your Body with Balls and Bands, Denise Austin, pg 5-7

51. 101 Ways to Work Out on the Ball: Sculpt Your Ideal Body with Pilates, Yoga, Elizabeth Gillies, pg 11

53. How to Buy a Ball, Aug 2008, Prevention Magazine Page 119

54. Weight Training for Women: Step-by-Step Exercises for Weight Loss, Body Shaping, and Good Health, by Leah Garcia, pg 30

55. Women's Health Jun 2006, Winning Workouts, by Katie Neitz, pg 74

56. The Complete Guide to Bodyweight Training, Kesh Patel, pg 14

57, 62. Men's Health Sep 2006, Scott Quill, pg 60

58-59. The Athlete's Book of Home Remedies, Jordan Metzl, pg 24

60. Runner's World Feb 2007, pg 32

61. Strength Training for Fat Loss, Nick Tumminello, page 168

63. The About.Com Guide to Getting in Shape: Simple and Fun Exercises to Help You Look and Feel Your Best (2007) By Paige Waehner, pg 77

64, 71. Your Body Is Your Barbell, BJ Gaddour, pg 4

65-70. Bodyweight Strength Training Anatomy, Bret Contreras, pg 168-169

72, 77, 79. Pilates For Dummies, Ellie Herman

73. The Core Connection, Chris Robinson, pg 6

74, 76, 78. Pilates for Every Body: Strengthen, Lengthen, and Tone, Denise Austin, pg 6

75. The Everything Wedding Workout Book, Shirley Archer, Andrea Mattei, pg 211

80, 82. Yoga Journal May 2001, On Your Knees by Julie Gudmestad, pg 141

81. Yoga Journal Mar-Apr 2000, Are You Weak in the Knees, By Dimity McDowell, pg 67-68

83. The Women's Health Big Book of Yoga, by Kathryn Budig, pg 257

84. Fitness After 40: How to Stay Strong at Any Age, by Vonda WRIGHT M.D., pg 108

85. Runner's World May 2007, page 92

86-87. Yoga Journal Jan-Feb 2004, Thighs Matter by Julie Gudmestad, pg 108

88. Say Goodbye to Knee Pain, By Marian Betancourt, Jo Hannafin, page 191

89. Heath - Best Supplements, by Erin Hobday, Men's Health Jul 2006, page 129

90. The Knee Crisis Handbook: Understanding Pain, Preventing Trauma by Brian Halpern, page 60

91-92. Ask are Healthy Joint Expert, Prevention Aug 2008, pg 8

93-94. The Knee Crisis Handbook: Understanding Pain, Preventing Trauma by Brian Halpern, page 61, 66

95-96. The Everything Pregnancy Fitness, Robin Elise Weiss, pg 153

98, 101. The Everything Guide to Pregnancy Nutrition & Health, Britt Brandon, pg 165-166

99-100. Nine Months Strong: Shaping Up for Labor and Delivery and the Toughest Physical Day of Your Life, by By Karen Bridson and Karin Blakemore

Printed in Great Britain
by Amazon